Magnesium:
The Miracle Mineral

Sandra Cabot MD

"You won't believe the DIFFERENCE it makes to your HEALTH and your SEX LIFE!"

Magnesium: The Miracle Mineral

Copyright © 2004 Dr Sandra Cabot
Edited and reprinted for the USA 2011

published by

SCB Inc. - United States of America
PO Box 5070 Glendale AZ USA 85312
Phone 623 334 3232

www.liverdoctor.com
www.weightcontroldoctor.com
www.sandracabot.com

ISBN: 978-0-982-93364-0

1) Magnesium 2) Stress 3) Depression 4) Anxiety 5) Heart Disease 6) High Blood Pressure 7) Magnesium the great relaxer 8) Erectile Dysfunction

Disclaimer - The suggestions, ideas and treatments described in this book must not replace the care and direct supervision of a trained health care professional. All problems and concerns regarding your health require medical supervision by a medical doctor. If you have any pre-existing medical disorders, you must consult your own doctor before following the suggestions in this book. If you are taking any prescribed medications, you should check with your own doctor before using the recommendations in this book.

About the Author

Dr Sandra Cabot MBBS, DRCOG, is a medical doctor who has extensive clinical experience in holistic medicine. Her offices are situated in Sydney, Australia and Phoenix, Arizona.

Dr Sandra Cabot began studying nutritional medicine while she was a medical student and has been a pioneer in the field of nutritional medicine. She graduated in medicine with honours from the University of Adelaide, South Australia in 1975. During the 1980s Dr Cabot worked as a volunteer in the largest missionary Christian hospital in India, tending to the poor indigenous women. Dr Sandra Cabot is a volunteer Angel Flight Pilot. See www.sandracabot.com

Other Books by Dr Cabot

Fatty Liver - You Can Reverse It

Liver Cleansing Diet

Healthy Liver and Bowel Book

Bird Flu - Your Survival Guide

Body Shaping Diet

Boost Your Energy

Cholesterol: The Real Truth

The Ultimate Detox

Help for Depression and Anxiety

Infertility - The Hidden Causes

Hormones - Don't Let Them Ruin Your Life

Hormone Replacement - The Real Truth

Raw Juices Can Save Your Life

Diabetes Type 2: You Can Reverse it Naturally

Alzheimer's - What you Must Know to Protect your Brain

Want to Lose Weight but Hooked on Food?

Your Thyroid Problems Solved

Can't Lose Weight - Unlock the Secrets that Keep you Fat

Infertility -the hidden causes

Tired of Not Sleeping? Wholistic Program for a Good Night Sleep

Her free health magazines are available online at www.liverdoctor.com

Dr Cabot founded the National Health Advisory Service in 1981, as a non-government funded service. This service has provided telephone and internet advice for people of all ages and has been helping people to find holistic solutions to their health problems for over 25 years. The Health Advisory Service helps to raise money for women's refuges and fire fighters in New South Wales.

For more information phone Dr Cabot's Health Lines
USA 623 334 3232 - Australia 02 4655 8855
or email ehelp@liverdoctor.com

I will let you in on a little secret

I have been recommending magnesium supplements for many years to help reduce a wide range of symptoms, which you will learn about in the following pages of this book. I have been recommending it to quite a few male patients to help them with high blood pressure, tremor, racing heart beat, stress and much more.

It was not until 2004 that I learnt of a surprising benefit, or you could even say, side effect of magnesium in males!

My male patients kept on thanking me for prescribing magnesium to them telling me it was absolutely terrific in every way and they could not believe the difference it had made in their lives. I mean I knew magnesium was a miracle for health, but I had not realised it was this good!

Finally I asked a couple of the guys I also knew as friends as well as patients, why they were so "over the moon" about the magnesium supplement that I had prescribed for them. They said "Well Sandra, I am a new man in the bedroom" and "I am 21 again" and I got it!

Magnesium was acting as a natural form of "Viagra" and they were trying to let me know!

Well it's not really surprising that magnesium can improve sexual performance in men because it acts as a "vasodilator" which means it dilates blood vessels and thus increases the circulation of blood through the blood vessles. Thus the function of the organs supplied by the blood vessels is enhanced.

Magnesium acts as a vasodilator because it relaxes the muscles in the arteries and this produces other beneficial effects such as improved circulation to the limbs (no more cold feet and hands!) and improved circulation to the brain (less migraines and better memory)

To gain the benefits of magnesium as a vasodilator, you need to take it regularly at least once a day.

So here's to your health and your love life!

Sandra Cabot

Sandra Cabot MD

Contents

Chapter 4

Chapter 5

Chapter 6

Chapter 7

Magnesium: The Miracle Mineral

Introduction

When it comes to improving health and living a healthy lifestyle, there are many people in today's world who expend their energy hoping for an effortless shortcut . . . a magic potion, so to speak, or more accurately, a magic pill. For reasons of their own they'd rather not invest the effort it takes to exercise or diet or pursue any of the other positive lifestyle changes that can prevent a lot of the most common medical conditions – and on one level I can understand why. Exercise is time consuming. Sacrifice is definitely no fun.

Instead, if given the choice, many people would undoubtedly opt for a pill to counteract the heart-damaging effects of poor eating habits, or to replace physical activity as a way of reducing diabetic complications, or to stave off irritability, do away with tension headaches or eliminate a host of other unpleasant conditions.

As anyone who has read any of my books knows, I am a very strong proponent of a healthy lifestyle that includes proper diet, exercise and a holistic approach to life. I will personally follow this lifestyle no matter what, and would under any and all circumstances recommend that everyone else do the same.

But if there were a mineral – a mineral found in your body and one that your health requires – that came in a pill/supplement form and provided all of the health benefits I previously mentioned, plus many more to boot, I would certainly take it. Wouldn't you?

Well, guess what? There is such a mineral and it is available over the counter – no prescription needed – in practically every health food store and pharmacy in the world.

As a medical doctor, I'm very much aware that prescription medications can treat, and even prevent, many of our most common health problems. I'm also aware that a lot of these medications are expensive, are often effective for just a single condition, can sometimes cause side effects that are worse than the health problems they control, and may require repeat visits to the doctor to ensure the dosage is correct.

Not that I'm against prescription medications – nothing could be further from the truth. Some man-made drugs, such as anti-hypertensive drugs and anti-depressant drugs for example, can truly work miracles, and have made the world a much healthier place. Still, there is always the cost and the side effects to consider, along with the fact that a prescription drug that works well for one person may not work quite as well for the next. And let's not forget the holistic approach. Given the choice between a man-made remedy and one found in nature, I'll always choose to follow the natural path – as long as the end result is the same or better.

To have a mineral found in nature, a mineral your body needs, a mineral that is easily and cheaply available (in pill or powder form) and known to be useful in treating or preventing dozens of medical conditions – to me, that sounds like a dream come true.

In this case, the dream has a name: magnesium.

Magnesium is a white mineral element found in the body's soft tissues, muscles and bones and, to some extent, in the body fluids. It is a naturally occurring element on earth, being extracted from ground water and seawater. The human body contains approximately 25 grams (just under 1 ounce) of magnesium, most of which is stored in the bones.

Magnesium is essential for hundreds of chemical reactions that take place in the body every second, with recent findings also indicating that it offers a wide range of important health-promoting benefits, including:

- Preventing muscle cramps
- Preventing heart disease
- Helping the body produce and use insulin
- Promoting strong bones and teeth
- Regulating heart rhythm

- Reducing high blood pressure
- Preventing the build up of excess calcium in the arteries, kidneys and soft tissues
- Reducing asthma
- Preventing headaches, including migraine
- Reducing chronic fatigue
- Reducing stress and anxiety
- Promoting a deep restful sleep
- Reducing epileptic convulsions
- Reducing the development of kidney stones
- Optimizing the performance of professional athletes
- Improving sexual performance in men

Honestly, the list of conditions that can be helped by magnesium goes on and on, yet a surprisingly large number of adults and children are magnesium deficient. And unfortunately, this widespread deficiency often remains undiagnosed by medical science because many doctors are not trained at university to recognize the symptoms of deficiency and laboratory testing for magnesium levels is not a commonly ordered test.

How serious is the problem of magnesium deficiency?

In one study that analyzed the diets of 564 adults, both male and female, the average intake of magnesium was less than two-thirds of the recommended daily allowance (RDA) for men and less than 50 percent of the RDA for women. Add to this the fact that, in my professional opinion, the RDA falls significantly short of the amount of magnesium you should actually be consuming, and you can see the potential size and scope of the magnesium deficiency problem.

The current RDA, by the way, is between 300 and 400 milligrams (mg) a day, depending on your sex and age.

Under optimal circumstances, a well-balanced diet that contains lots of nuts, fruits, vegetables and whole grains should provide the minimum RDA of magnesium. Unfortunately, in most parts of the world and for most people, optimal circumstances don't exist. Modern, chemical-rich fertilizers alter the ability of plants to draw magnesium from the soil. Food processing further removes magnesium. High-carbohydrate and refined processed diets increase the need for magnesium, as does stress. Dieting can significantly reduce magnesium intake.

In other words, many of the activities common to modern daily living can have a serious impact on your magnesium levels, and set you up for any number of potentially serious medical conditions.

For these reasons, I've researched and written **Magnesium: The Miracle Mineral.** It will set the record straight on the value of magnesium and its ability to help you fend off multiple illnesses.

In the following pages, you'll read about the symptoms of magnesium deficiency, learn of the many medical problems a deficiency can cause, discover the best sources of magnesium, be alerted to safety issues, find recommended daily dosages . . and much, much more.

If you suffer with persistent and/or mysterious health problems, there is a good chance that **Magnesium: The Miracle Mineral** can and will change your life for the better – and the healthier. Even if you are already in better-than-average health with no apparent physical or mental issues, there's still a very good chance that increasing your magnesium intake will boost your health to the next highest level.

If you've been looking for that magic pill I mentioned earlier, then it's fair to say that your search is now over. You've found the pot of gold at the end of the good health rainbow, and it's filled with magnesium.

Magnesium:
The Miracle Mineral

Chapter 1
Understanding Magnesium

If you're not already at least partially convinced that magnesium – a very common, everyday nutrient – can prevent, treat and potentially reverse a wide range of health-related problems, both physical and mental, then this is a must-read chapter for you. Why?

Not to date myself, but I've been a medical doctor for a relatively long time. In all my years of practice, I've not come across any other nutrient – or any prescription medication, for that matter – that is magnesium's equal for the number of different ways it can improve your health and well being.

It's my professional opinion that one reason you don't hear more about this wonder nutrient . . . and the main reason it's not promoted more strongly by the pharmaceutical community . . . is that magnesium is not a drug that can be patented. This takes away the profit incentive, which I'm sorry to say also takes away the desire of most major drug companies to both study and promote magnesium.

You may think this is a harsh judgment. But given the negative impact of widespread magnesium deficiency on the health of millions of people and the corresponding lack of concern by the majority of mainstream drug researchers and manufacturers, it is also a fair comment. When it comes to my health and yours, "fair" is always going to be more important to me than "harsh."

In the Introduction to Magnesium: The Miracle Mineral, I gave you a dictionary definition of magnesium. At this point, I could easily offer up reams of additional scientific descriptions (most of them really technical) of this alkaline macromineral and what it does... but in order to keep you alert and paying attention, let me just reiterate that magnesium is needed by every cell in your body and is responsible for the correct metabolic (chemical changes in cells through which energy is provided for vital activities) function of more than 300 – and possibly as many as 350 – enzymes. (Enzymes are the complex proteins produced by your body's cells.)

Research coming out of Europe indicates that magnesium likewise plays a key role in the release of many hormones and nutrients, and that it protects cells from heavy metals such as mercury and lead. Magnesium deficiency may contribute to learning disorders and Attention Deficit Disorder in children.

Magnesium is also required for such things as ion transport across cell membranes (ions are electrically charged minerals) and the synthesis of essential molecules. The magnesium molecule stabilizes the electrical potential that exists across the cell membrane and this is vitally important for preventing unwanted electrical discharges in body tissues. Unwanted electrical discharges could result in an epileptic fit or panic attack (if they occurred in the brain) or a fatal heart arrhythmia if they occurred in the heart muscle.

But again, this type of scientific data can be too academic, and if my years of treating patients and writing books has taught me anything, it's that most people will be more interested about the role of magnesium in, say, reducing the risk of heart disease or preventing anxiety than how it is "required by the adenosine triphosphate synthesizing protein in mitochondria."

Magnesium, by the way, can help prevent heart disease and anxiety, but before we head any further in that direction, I'd like to address in a little more depth the growing magnesium deficiency in a large proportion of the world's population. This occurs in countries of all prosperity levels, from the very richest to the absolute poorest.

One thing I've noticed in researching this subject is that some medical professionals do not believe there's a magnesium deficiency crisis. In fact, they will tell you that while surveys might indicate many people in even the most developed countries do not receive the recommended daily minimum amount, magnesium deficiency is still rarely recognized.

There are a number of reasons I don't agree with this, beginning with surveys that suggest at least four out of every 10 people – or 40 percent of the population – are magnesium deficient. I've seen statistics that show Germans have an average intake of only 67 percent of the RDA (recommended daily allowance) of magnesium, while the Japanese lag even farther behind at 53 percent.

Other countries do better, and Australia is one of the best, with one survey showing that 98 percent of Australians reach the RDI (recommended daily intake) for magnesium. It should be noted, however, that Australia's RDI is but 90 percent of the RDA used in the United States and other countries, which means there is still room for significant deficiency. And as I've said before – I don't believe that either the RDA or the RDI provides a sufficient amount of magnesium to meet your body's total needs, especially if you are under stress or are a high performing individual.

Traditionally, most people get magnesium only from the various foods they eat, and sometimes from their drinking water. In the United States, two fairly recent national surveys indicated that the diets of "most adult men and women do not provide the recommended amounts of magnesium." And it was suggested that the problem is even worse in adults over age 70.

I've seen other surveys that put the overall deficiency rate as high as 75 or 80 percent – again showing that when it comes to magnesium deficiency, you will most certainly find a difference of opinion.

Tests for Magnesium

Contributing to the statistical discrepancies in the incidence of magnesium deficiency is the fact that there really isn't a single, reliable laboratory test that can accurately identify a lack of total body magnesium. Only 1 percent of your body's magnesium, for example, is found in the blood – so a test to measure blood levels of magnesium is not going to be very definitive in terms of uncovering a possible overall deficiency. Doctors more commonly do a test called "red blood cell magnesium", which measures the amount of magnesium inside the red blood cells; this test is more reliable than whole blood magnesium, but is still not an accurate reflection of total body magnesium levels. This is easy to understand because as much as 60 percent of all the magnesium in your body is found in your bones, another 25 percent or so is found in muscle, and the remainder – minus the one percent found in the blood – is located inside your cells. It would be more accurate to take a sample (biopsy) of the bone or muscle and test its magnesium level – but I'm sure you would not want such an invasive and painful test!

Normal Ranges of Magnesium in blood and urine tests

Specimen	Values	Units (metric)
Whole Blood	1.1 - 1.9	mmol/L
Red Blood Cells	1.7 - 2.8	mmol/L
24hr Urine	2.5 - 6.3	mmol/24hr
Urine	2 - 8	mmol/L

Taken from ARL Laboratories data base

L = Liter (33.8oz)

mmol = millimoles

Another test that can be used to measure magnesium status is called a "loading test." It works like this: Urine is tested over a 24-hour period to get a baseline measurement of its magnesium content. Then, the patient is given a "load" of magnesium and the 24-hour urine test is repeated.

If the magnesium excretion is high, a deficiency is unlikely, as your body will get rid of what it doesn't need. If, in turn, magnesium excretion is low, this means a deficiency is possible because your body is retaining the bulk of the extra magnesium.

Note, please, that the two key words used to describe the results of this test are "unlikely" and "possible" – meaning that the results are nothing on which you would want to bet your life … or your health.

Yet another test, the Blood Ionized Magnesium Test, was developed by veteran magnesium researchers Drs. Bella and Burton Altura to specifically identify magnesium ions. The accuracy of this test has "been confirmed countless times with sensitive digital imaging microscopy, atomic absorption spectroscopy and the magnesium fluorescent probe." Unfortunately, the Altura's test is not readily available to the vast majority of the world's population – so that alone somewhat decreases its value.

Finally, I've also seen some questionnaires that assign points to such things as how often you eat foods high in magnesium (such as fresh vegetables, nuts, whole grain breads and cereals), and whether or not you have high blood pressure, high cholesterol or a family history of heart disease. Totalling your points will give you an idea of your risk for magnesium deficiency. Unfortunately, this is just a general guide and the results are probably not as accurate as you'd like and certainly not as accurate as a definitive medical test – if only one existed.

In addition to the almost universal lack of precision in magnesium testing, I've found, too, that research into how magnesium affects the human body has for years been stymied by either a lack of interest that relates back to the profit motive, or by a lack of imaginative technology.

We, as doctors and scientists, are somewhat behind the curve when it comes to scientifically tracking the many ways in which magnesium can improve your state of health, along with your state of mind.

So, in light of this somewhat disheartening information, you're probably asking yourself, *"What's the most accurate way of determining a magnesium deficiency"?*

My answer is that you essentially have two choices:

1. There are laboratory-type tests and questionnaires that at best either offer "semi-conclusive" results or are offered on a relatively small scale in a limited number of locations.

2. There are a large number of magnesium deficiency signs, symptoms and conditions that are usually very accurate in pointing to a magnesium problem - see page 18.

Personally, I'm inclined at present to rely most heavily on the signs and symptoms option, and will continue to do so until I'm convinced that medical science, as regards magnesium deficiency, has caught up with common sense.

Causes of Magnesium Deficiency

Many times, a magnesium deficiency can be caused by medical conditions that affect the body's ability to handle magnesium, or by certain substances that have a negative effect on the nutrient.

These include:

- Gastrointestinal diseases that cause poor absorption of magnesium or a loss of magnesium through diarrhea and vomiting.

- Treatment with diuretics (water or fluid tablets), which increases the loss of magnesium in urine. The diuretic drugs most likely to cause magnesium loss are known as loop and thiazide diuretics (e.g. lasix and hydrochlorthiazide).

- Excess use of laxatives, causing loose stools or diarrhea.

- Alcohol abuse, because alcohol increases urinary excretion of magnesium. Also, many alcoholics will substitute alcohol for food, further lowering their magnesium levels by restricting intake.

- Certain chemotherapy medicines (such as cisplatin) used to treat cancer can increase loss of magnesium in the urine

- Certain antibiotics (such as amphotericin, gentamicin, and tetracyclines) may increase urinary loss of magnesium and reduce magnesium absorption.

- People with diabetes who don't control their blood sugar levels. Diabetes also results in a greater loss of magnesium in the urine.

- Frequent or severe vomiting. Occasional vomiting, in and of itself, generally won't lead to a magnesium problem.

- Chronically low blood levels of the mineral potassium, which at times indicate an underlying problem with magnesium deficiency.

- Poor absorption of dietary fat, which can be caused by intestinal surgery or infection or celiac disease, as well as inflammatory bowel disease such as Crohn's disease.

- Dieting, especially fad diets, will generally reduce your daily intake of magnesium.

In addition, age could also be a factor in magnesium deficiency, with people over 70 oftentimes having relatively low dietary intakes of magnesium.

Other known or suspected reasons for having less than desirable levels of magnesium are:

- Long term use of drugs to suppress the production of hydrochloric acid from the stomach (eg. proton pump inhibitors or H2 receptor antagonists) These drugs can produce significant deficiencies of magnesium.
- Eating too many carbohydrates, especially white sugar and white flour
- Chronic pain
- Drinking too much coffee
- Drinking too much alcohol
- Extreme physical training
- High doses of zinc in supplement form
- A sudden and/or large increase of fiber in the diet
- Fizzy soft drinks, either diet colas or those high in sugar
- High salt intake
- Physical stress
- Mental stress, anxiety and depression
- Excessive perspiration
- Recreational drug use; e.g. amphetamines and cocaine

What this information tells us, for instance, is that if you are a long-distance runner with a fondness for coffee, who eats a lot of sugar and is under a lot of pressure at work, then you could very well have a significant or even severe magnesium deficiency. The same holds true if you have chronic stomach problems and take antacids, are often dieting, or suffer with diabetes.

What Are the Symptoms of Magnesium Deficiency?

But what if none of the conditions I've mentioned above really apply to you? You could still have a magnesium deficiency, but how would you know? Well, there are a number of different symptoms that can indicate a deficiency, but before I list them it is important to mention that many of these symptoms could also be indicative of another condition that's potentially much more serious, at least in the short term, than a low level of magnesium.

So, if you experience one or more of the following symptoms, please don't self diagnose and just assume the problem is related to a magnesium deficiency. Talk to your doctor or other healthcare provider, and make sure that what you may think is a problem with magnesium is not actually caused by something else.

Here is a list of the common and possible symptoms of magnesium deficiency:

- High blood pressure
- Heart palpitations (irregular heart beat)
- Rapid heart beat (racing pulse or tachycardia)
- Cold hands and feet
- Mental confusion
- Anxiety
- Panic attacks
- Kidney stones
- Shortness of breath
- Poor digestion and constipation
- Irritable bowel syndrome
- Insomnia
- Depression
- Vertigo or dizziness
- Headaches, especially migraine, vascular or tension headaches
- Muscular aches and pains
- Low exercise tolerance
- Muscle twitches, spasms and cramps
- Irritability
- Increase in epileptic convulsions
- Inability to control epilepsy with drugs
- Unstable blood sugar levels and cravings for sugar
- Frequent sports injuries
- Fibromyalgia

The problem with providing a list of symptoms such as these is that you're bound to leave one or more out, as different individuals can have a different physical or mental response to a low level of magnesium. While this is a good list in the sense that it covers most of the more common symptoms, don't automatically dismiss other symptoms as being unrelated to magnesium.

As you continue to read Magnesium: The Miracle Mineral, you'll learn more about the various foods and herbs that provide a good supply of dietary magnesium.

I'll also discuss supplements, and you will find a lot of information on the many medical conditions that can result from magnesium deficiency. Collectively, these facts and figures should help give you an even better idea of where you stand in regard to your body's magnesium content, and what you can do to make sure you maintain a healthy magnesium level.

Magnesium:
The Miracle Mineral

Chapter 2

Health Problems helped by Magnesium - A to C

With each passing year, more and more studies are validating magnesium as beneficial in the prevention of a wide range of diseases and health problems. Yet millions of people worldwide remain in the dark, having little if any familiarity with this "miracle mineral" and the fact that every single cell in your body needs an adequate amount of magnesium if you plan on staying healthy, strong and energetic.

In a broad sense, a human body that's severely deficient in magnesium is similar to a car that is running exceedingly low on petrol; neither is going to carry you as far as you'll probably want to go.

Years of practising medicine, plus a long-time research interest in the benefits of magnesium, has allowed me to compile a list of moderate to severe health problems that can be attributed – in part, at least – to a magnesium deficiency.

There is still much research to be done into the overall effects of magnesium on human health. I'm a bit reluctant to list a health problem as being related to magnesium deficiency unless I've personally seen magnesium improve that problem or condition, or I've read research literature from a reputable source that convinces me that a low magnesium level is responsible for the problem/condition.

Hence, the list compiled for this book contains only 32 disorders, though I don't for a second doubt that with time and additional research it's a list that could be lengthened considerably.

But before we begin, **PLEASE NOTE** that if you suffer with any of these disorders, it's imperative that you seek professional medical attention. While taking a magnesium supplement or adding foods high in magnesium to your diet will provide many benefits, I'm not suggesting that treating any of these conditions on your own – and with magnesium alone – should or could ever take the place of a thorough plan of care worked out with your doctor or other healthcare provider.

Magnesium is beyond a doubt one key to a healthier life – not the only key, but certainly a most important one.

Adrenal Gland Exhaustion

The adrenal glands are two small glands; one is situated on top of each kidney. The adrenal glands are vitally important to health and wellbeing because they produce hormones that allow us to cope with stress, both physical and mental in origin.

The symptoms of adrenal gland exhaustion include:

- Fatigue, especially in the mornings, which can be severe and overwhelming
- Depression
- Increasing allergies
- Increasing inflammation in the body
- Low tolerance to physical and mental stress
- Dizziness and low blood pressure
- Low libido

The condition of adrenal gland exhaustion has become more common over the last decade for several reasons:

- People are more stressed
- People sleep less
- Magnesium deficiency is common
- Infections and toxins such as cigarettes, excess alcohol and sugar damage the adrenal glands

The function of the adrenal glands is highly dependent upon magnesium, which enables the cells in the adrenal glands to produce the energy they need to manufacture the steroid hormones (such as cortisol and sex hormones) and adrenalin.

I have found that most of my patients with adrenal gland dysfunction are very deficient in magnesium and antioxidants. It is easy to test the function of the adrenal glands with blood and urine tests; however, more subtle degrees of dysfunction are often missed with conventional tests.

If you have the symptoms of adrenal gland exhaustion, see your doctor for tests of adrenal function.

If you have persistent symptoms of adrenal gland exhaustion I recommend the following:

- Magnesium – 400 mg daily
- Selenium – 100 mcg daily
- Adrenal Plus Support Tablets (see page 96)
- Fish oil capsules – 2 capsules twice daily just before eating
- Raw juicing to boost antioxidants – use purple cabbage, ginger, parsley, spinach, apple, celery and orange.

Angina

Angina results from an insufficient supply of oxygen to the heart muscle, which in turn may cause a squeezing feeling or heavy pain in the front of your chest – pain that sometimes spreads to the left shoulder, left arm and up into the jaw. Generally, physical exertion and/or stress initiate an angina attack, because they increase the heart's need for oxygen. Angina is most often the result of atherosclerosis – the build-up of cholesterol-containing plaque inside the coronary arteries that narrows the arteries and reduces the flow of blood to the heart muscle. There is also a second and less common type of angina – Prinzmetal's variant angina – which is caused by a spasm in one or more coronary arteries. This type of angina is most likely to occur when you are resting or stressed.

A number of studies over the past 20 years or so have shown that magnesium is very important in preventing or reducing the severity of angina, with some reports going so far as to suggest that in most people magnesium should be the treatment of choice for Prinzmetal's variant. Magnesium reduces spasms in the coronary arteries, improves delivery of oxygen to the heart muscle by relaxing and opening up the coronary arteries, and improves production of energy within the heart muscle. In essence, magnesium enables muscles in your coronary arteries – and all other arteries, for that matter – to relax. And you can be sure that a relaxed artery is more effective in delivering oxygenated blood than an artery that's constricted.

One of the world's foremost experts on the health benefits of magnesium has said that "the normal constriction and dilation of the arteries ... is influenced by hormones, the secretion of which is controlled by the amount of magnesium present." In other words, if you want a healthy heart and don't care to experience the pain and discomfort of angina, you would be wise to get an adequate amount of magnesium on a daily basis.

Anxiety Disorder

Anxiety, which is defined as "an unpleasant emotional state

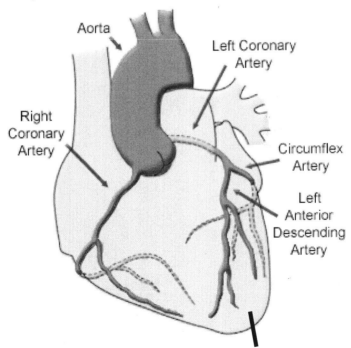

The heart muscle is supplied with oxygenated blood
from the coronary arteries

ranging from mild unease to intense fear", is a normal part of everyday life for millions of people.

All age groups are affected, with the general exception of the very young. And to clarify, anxiety differs from fear in that anxiety most often has no realistic or clear-cut cause, while fear is usually your response to an actual danger.

Though a little anxiety is to be expected from time to time in everyone but the exceptionally calm – and some hold the opinion that a low level of anxiety may even be healthy because it can prompt you to act or react when you might otherwise not – excessive anxiety can and does lead to significant mental and physical problems.

Currently, medical science recognizes half-a-dozen anxiety disorders, which can be overwhelming and lead to irrational and involuntary fears of ordinary situations, places or objects. Panic disorder is one, along with generalized anxiety disorder, obsessive-compulsive disorder (OCD), post-traumatic stress disorder (PTSD), social anxiety disorder, and a wide range of specific phobias. I assure you that none of these disorders is in the least bit pleasant, and all can be accompanied by physical symptoms that run the full spectrum, from trembling and dizziness, to chest pains, muscle tension and inability to concentrate, to sweating and rapid heartbeat.

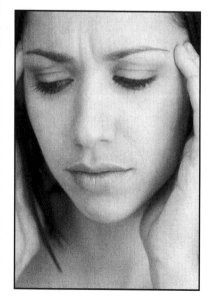

Research into the relationship between a magnesium deficiency and anxiety disorders is still in its infancy – which is also the case with many of the conditions that follow. Still, I have found that magnesium is very helpful in reducing anxiety, especially in highly stressed people who find it hard to relax.

One researcher has observed decreased levels of nervousness in patients supplemented with magnesium, while a different investigation found that post-surgical patients given intravenous magnesium reported less anxiety.

Also, high lactic acid levels are thought by some experts to be an underlying factor in anxiety. Magnesium deficiency is one of the factors that may be responsible if your lactic acid is elevated.

Like other medical professionals, I sometimes call magnesium the "great relaxer." It not only relaxes the muscles, but it also relaxes the entire nervous system – helping you feel calmer and less stressed when you are under a lot of pressure or when anxiety otherwise invades your everyday life.

Arrhythmia of the heart

A healthy and properly functioning heart beats in a regular rhythm and at a rate that is directly related to your body's activity level. When your heartbeat gets out of synch – when it beats too fast, or too slow or with an irregular rhythm – this is a condition known as arrhythmia.

Many changes in heartbeat are minor and do not require medical treatment, while others are more serious and can increase your risk of a deadly heart attack or stroke. If you feel your heart skipping a beat or beating in an unusual or irregular manner, or if you feel a fluttering in your chest, please seek immediate help. Only a qualified medical professional can determine the seriousness of an arrhythmia.

Having said that, it is no secret in the medical community that a significant number of heart rhythm disorders are related to a low or insufficient level of magnesium in the heart muscle. Several published reports say magnesium was first shown to have value in treating arrhythmia as far back as 1935. Clinical studies over the succeeding years have indicated that magnesium may benefit several different types of arrhythmia, including atrial fibrillation, ventricular premature contractions, ventricular tachycardia and ventricular arrhythmias. The latter start in the lower chambers of the heart and can be life threatening.

In one study of more than 230 people with frequent heart

arrhythmias, the abnormal rhythms dropped "significantly" within a three-week period after the participants increased the amount of magnesium and potassium in their diets. It is believed that magnesium depletion within the heart muscle is often associated with potassium depletion too.

Another study found that taking a magnesium supplement may provide considerable benefits to people suffering with new-onset atrial fibrillation (a malfunction in the upper chambers of the heart). The prescription drug of choice for this condition is digoxin, though it is largely ineffective in restoring proper heart rhythm. When digoxin and magnesium were given together, however, 60 percent of patients reverted to a normal heart rhythm. In a group that received digoxin only, the figure was 38 percent. The results of this study strongly indicate that magnesium either greatly improves the efficiency of digoxin or offers significant benefits on its own. If you ever experience an irregular heartbeat, talk to your doctor about the wisdom of taking a magnesium supplement on a regular basis.

Arthritis

Arthritis, in the simplest of terms, is nothing more than inflammation of a joint. The most common form of arthritis is osteoarthritis, which is characterized by a loss of function in a joint and a loss of cartilage (the shock-absorbing tissue between joints). In osteoarthritis, the damage basically comes as a result of years of wear and tear on the joint and this is worsened by repeated injuries. Arthritis can also be caused by gout or auto-immune inflammation, as seen in rheumatoid arthritis.

Several studies have shown that a diet rich in vegetables – which, if properly planned, will also be a diet rich in magnesium – has a role in the management of joint diseases. Articular cartilage, or cartilage in the joints, is critically dependent upon nutrients such as glucose, vitamins, particularly vitamin C, and essential trace elements such as magnesium. In addition, I've seen first hand in my own practice that maintaining an adequate level of magnesium can offer significant benefits to patients with joint disorders, including those of you with osteoarthritis.

In arthritis patients we must do two things:

1. **Strengthen the bones and cartilage** with the minerals calcium, magnesium, zinc, boron, silica and manganese. Vitamin D supplements are usually required in a dose of 1000 to 4000 units daily. Glucosamine supports cartilage.

2. **Reduce inflammation** with omega 3 fatty acids from fish oil and flaxseed oil and the minerals copper and selenium.

Asthma

At some point in our lives, most all of us have had a friend or a family member who suffered with the wheezing, the coughing, the chest congestion and the shortness of breath that characterizes asthma. It's not a pleasant condition and, in fact, under the right circumstances, asthma can even kill you. Basically, asthma is an allergic disorder characterized by spasms in the airway (bronchial tubes), swelling of the mucous lining of the bronchial tubes and the excessive production of mucous.

Avoiding the airborne and food-related allergens that can lead to an asthma attack is a good first step in any prevention plan, but medical scientists have known for nearly 100 years that magnesium relaxes bronchial muscles. By helping these muscles to relax and allowing the lung's airways to expand, magnesium can help relieve the shortness of breath and wheezing characteristic of asthma. Today, giving magnesium intravenously is widely recognized as an effective way to halt an acute asthma attack. And reports from different countries around the world have shown or indicated that combining magnesium with conventional medical therapies can oftentimes make those therapies more effective in preventing asthma attacks.

Overall, the evidence is pretty overwhelming: a lack of magnesium is often a major contributor to asthma or asthma-like conditions, and magnesium has a role alongside more conventional therapies in treating patients with asthma. In light of this information, common sense tells me that it is foolish to wait until an asthma attack occurs before administering magnesium.

If you are someone who suffers with asthma, I'd recommend that in conjunction with your prescribed medications you follow a diet rich in magnesium-laden foods or take a daily magnesium supplement, or both. Why take a chance on suffering when that suffering could very possibly be avoided?

Other important avoidance strategies against asthma and respiratory infections include taking fish oil, vitamin C and selenium supplements.

Atherosclerosis

Atherosclerosis is popularly known as "hardening of the arteries."

It is basically a condition that's caused by the build-up of plaque (calcium deposits and cholesterol) inside the lining of the arteries. This causes the arteries to gradually become narrower and the flow of blood is restricted.

For these reasons, atherosclerosis is the starting point for many common circulatory problems such as a reduced blood flow to the heart, brain, various body organs and limbs.

In my research, I've discovered a number of studies that link hardening of the arteries to a magnesium deficiency. One of the

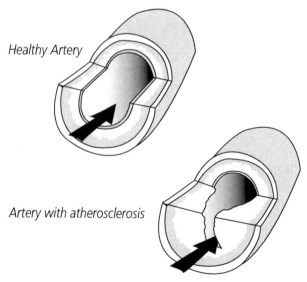

Healthy Artery

Artery with atherosclerosis

earliest dates back to 1958 in South Africa, where atherosclerotic heart disease was practically unknown in Bantu tribesmen – yet was very common in their white neighbors. It was found that, on average, the level of magnesium in the Bantu's blood was 11 percent higher than in the blood of the white South Africans. Also, a variety of accumulated data has shown that a magnesium deficiency can lead to atherosclerosis by increasing cholesterol concentrations and causing inflammation in the blood vessels. And laboratory tests are reportedly conclusive that low magnesium can set the stage for the formation of plaque in arteries.

Magnesium, which is relatively inexpensive and safe (more about the safety issue in Chapter 6), is not only considered very useful in preventing hardening of the arteries, it is also a good therapy for patients showing early signs of this disease. As one expert has stated unequivocally, "Magnesium keeps blood vessels soft and flexible, preventing a build-up of plaque within the arteries." Where coronary and cerebral arteries are concerned, "soft", "flexible" and "plaque free" are definitely all pluses. Another proven benefit is that magnesium is able to lower the amount of the protein called C-reactive protein that causes the inflammation in the arteries that leads to atherosclerosis.

Attention Deficit Disorder

Attention deficit disorder, or ADD, is a relatively current term that describes a variety of disorders in children and some adults, the most common probably being attention deficit hyperactivity disorder (ADHD). When I was a child, if you had an attention disorder you were commonly described as having "a hard time paying attention" or suffering from "a bad case of the wiggles." Or, perhaps your parents or teachers would have been concerned because "your mind was always somewhere else." Today, from a diagnostic standpoint, youngsters who are inattentive, impulsive, overly active, have a brief attention span or can't concentrate will likely be identified as having some form of ADD or ADHD.

It is just as likely that magnesium can help solve these problems. There are numerous studies to back up this opinion, but common sense also comes into play here. For instance, almost any list of the common symptoms of magnesium deficiency will include irritability, muscle twitches, confusion and difficulty concentrating – which are identical to classic symptoms of ADD. Is this just a coincidence? I don't think so!

In one study of 116 ADHD children between nine and 12 years of age, 95 percent – or 110 of the children – were magnesium deficient. Another study included 50 children with ADHD, all between the ages of seven and 12, who were divided into two groups of 25 children each. The children in one group received six months of magnesium supplementation; the children in the other group did not. The children who were given magnesium showed a "significant decrease in hyperactivity", as compared to those children who received no magnesium.

And this is just a minute sampling of the evidence. Recently, I typed "magnesium deficiency and attention deficit disorder" into a popular Internet search engine. I was rewarded with 120,000 hits! And no, obviously I did not read them all. However after all my research, I am totally convinced that if your child has any form of ADD, or is experiencing hyperactivity, then magnesium may be an answer to your prayers.

I would also suggest that you combine the magnesium supplement with sources of omega 3 essential fatty acids to support brain function and growth. Good sources are fish oil, oily fish and cold pressed flaxseed oil. Supplementation with the mineral iodine, as well as B vitamins, can also help brain development, intelligence and mood.

Bladder problems

Over the years I have come to see the diverse and often unexpected benefits of supplementing someone with magnesium; indeed the results have often amazed me!

For example, one of my patients who is well into her 70s suffered with poor sleep due to urinary frequency during the night – she would have to get up every few hours and hurry to the toilet to pass very small amounts of urine. This had troubled her for years and was only partially helped with estrogen therapy. Within two weeks of starting magnesium tablets in a dose of four tablets daily her bladder problem was completely relieved. She could not believe the difference this simple therapy had made to her sleep and thus her quality of life.

Bladder problems that can be helped by taking magnesium include:

- Recurrent cystitis
- Interstitial cystitis
- Nocturnal urinary frequency
- Wetting the bed in children
- Irritable bladder & incontinence

Interstitial cystitis is a chronic inflammation of the entire wall of the bladder affecting the muscle and mucous lining of the bladder wall. Its symptoms consist of pain in the area of the bladder above the pubic bone, urinary frequency and urgency and pain on passing urine. Sexual intercourse may also be painful in women afflicted with interstitial cystitis because the bladder is situated at the top of the vagina.

I have had several female patients who have found complete relief from the awful symptoms of interstitial cystitis by taking magnesium. Generally 400 mg daily is required.

I also highly recommend raw juicing in those who suffer with bladder inflammation and/or infection and good things to juice are ginger root, red onion, carrot, celery, mint, basil, citrus, green apples and cucumber. An estriol cream can be applied to the vulva to strengthen the pelvic floor and bladder. It is a pity that more doctors do not know about the tremendous benefits of supplemental magnesium for bladder problems. Magnesium should be tried before laser therapy to the bladder, which generally only has a temporary effect and can cause permanent bladder scarring.

Cardiomyopathy

I'm sure it has become apparent by now that a magnesium deficiency is definitely not good for your heart, and is in fact one of the leading causes of a number of heart-related diseases. One of these is cardiomyopathy, which is any disease of the heart muscle that lessens its ability to pump enough blood to meet your body's needs. The exact cause of cardiomyopathy may vary – it can be viral, metabolic, nutritional, toxic, auto-immune, genetic or even unknown – but the end result is going to be pretty much the same; some degree of heart failure.

Why is magnesium important in the prevention of cardiomyopathy? If the muscle cells in your heart don't receive adequate amounts of magnesium, they will lose the ability to produce the energy they need to contract and pump blood and its life-giving oxygen throughout your body. A heart that can't pump effectively is similar to a defective fuel pump in your car; both can lead to a loss of efficiency or power. If the problem is not corrected, there will come a day when the car – or your heart – will no longer function. There is "substantial experimental evidence" indicating that diets low in magnesium can be responsible for cardiomyopathy, while a number of different studies have shown that magnesium can and does improve heart function in patients who already have cardiomyopathy – and this is regardless of the specific cause.

In cases of cardiomyopathy I recommend the following:

- Magnesium, 400 mg elemental daily
- Selenomethionine, 200 mcg daily
- Vitamin C, 2000 mg daily
- Vitamin E, 500 I. U. twice daily
- Fish oil, 2000 mg twice daily just before food

Ask your doctor to check your thyroid function with a blood test and the concentration of iodine in your urine. Thyroid problems and/or iodine deficiency may worsen cardiomyopathy.

Cadiomyopathy is an auto-immune disease that may be triggered by gluten intolerance or viral infections.

Note: If you are taking blood thinning medication you will have to avoid large doses of vitamin E and fish oil. Do your heart – and yourself – a big favour. Make sure your daily magnesium intake is sufficient to stave off cardiomyopathy and other forms of cardiovascular disease.

Chronic Fatigue Syndrome

In over 30 years of practising medicine I have treated patients with an almost infinite number of diseases, conditions and syndromes – and I can honestly say that where the general public is concerned, chronic fatigue syndrome (CFS) is one of the most misunderstood. Though it has been affecting people for decades – more likely, centuries – and has been called so many different things that one doctor has described it as the "disease with a thousand names," CFS wasn't formally defined until the late 1980s. And it is much more serious, and much more involved, than just "being tired all the time."

People afflicted with chronic fatigue syndrome have varying combinations of symptoms, ranging from constant fatigue to loss of concentration, sore throat, emotional distress, low-grade fever, depression, swollen lymph nodes, stomach problems, headache, trouble sleeping, excessive fatigue after exercising, joint pain, and muscle weakness and pain. Regardless of your individual symptoms, however, a low level of magnesium may be a big part of the cause.

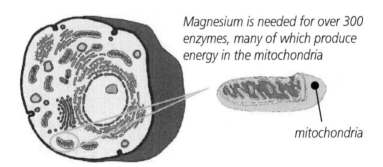

Magnesium is needed for over 300 enzymes, many of which produce energy in the mitochondria

mitochondria

A cell and its internal organs

In a clinical trial conducted in England, patients with CFS were divided into two groups. Patients in one group were given injections of magnesium every week for six weeks; in the other group, patients received injections of water. None of the patients were aware of which treatment they were receiving. At the end of the six-week period, 80 percent of the patients receiving magnesium reported higher energy levels, better emotional states and less pain, as compared to only 18 percent of patients in the group receiving water. Similar results have been obtained in other clinical trials, some dating back to the 1960s. Overall, the message is clear; a magnesium deficiency can lead to chronic fatigue and prevent recovery from it.

Congestive Heart Failure

Congestive heart failure (CHF), is caused by the heart's inability to effectively pump blood throughout the body. Fatigue, shortness of breath, a congestive cough, reduced ability to exercise and swelling of the ankles are the most common symptoms of heart failure.

Heart failure can be caused by:

- The long-term effects of high blood pressure
- Damage to the heart muscle, as the result of heart attack, atherosclerosis, diabetes, viral infection or cardiomyopathy
- A damaged heart valve
- Lung diseases
- Obesity

Congestive heart failure is very common – it affects an estimated one out of every 100 people in many developed countries. My research indicates that the vast majority of these people are likely to be deficient in magnesium.

Often, this deficiency is caused by a poor diet – the same sort of diet that leads to heart disease in the first place. At the same time, many CHF patients may experience magnesium deficiencies as a result of increased urinary excretion – as a consequence of prescribed diuretic drugs and/or digoxin therapy prescribed to treat heart failure.

In one study of congestive heart failure patients, those who tested normal for levels of magnesium had one and two year survival rates of 71 percent and 61 percent, respectively. Patients with low magnesium levels had survival rates of only 45 percent and 42 percent respectively. If something as affordable and as easily obtainable as magnesium can improve the survival rate of CHF patients by 20 percent or more, I would say that everyone –

especially people with a family history of heart disease – should be eating magnesium-rich foods and taking a magnesium supplement, and that's each and every day.

Constipation

Constipation is the term used to describe a lack of regular bowel actions. In addition, the stools are often hard and difficult to pass. Constipation can be caused by a diet lacking in fiber, a lack of water, stress, a lack of exercise or an enlarged redundant bowel. Fortunately, magnesium has proven to be a good antidote to constipation, so much so, in fact, that some people with expertise in the field have even taken to calling magnesium "nature's laxative."

For one thing, magnesium helps prevent constipation by relaxing the muscles in the walls of your colon. Spasm in these muscles can occur when you are under a lot of stress, when anxiety strikes or if you have inflammation in the bowel. Spasm of the bowel muscle can occur intermittently, leading to abdominal cramps, bloating, gas and irregular bowel actions that vary from constipation to diarrhea – this is called irritable bowel syndrome (IBS).

Magnesium also regulates and keeps the bowels alkaline; this reduces gas production in the intestines (everything from the oesophagus down through the stomach, intestines and colon). What a simple and safe remedy for the embarrassing problem of intestinal flatulence. Combine the magnesium supplement with peppermint oil capsules to get relief from irritable bowel syndrome.

The constipation/magnesium research study, that's probably referred to more than any other study, involved 64 people aged 65 years and older. This study showed that magnesium is even more effective at providing constipation relief than a bulk-laxative.

And – ready for some more good news? – unlike many popular over-the-counter laxatives, magnesium does not create a laxative dependency.

Many people with constipation and/or irritable bowel syndrome find that magnesium powder works better than magnesium tablets, especially in an ultrapotent form combined with the amino acid taurine. See page 96.

For more information on bowel problems see my book *The Healthy Liver and Bowel Book*.

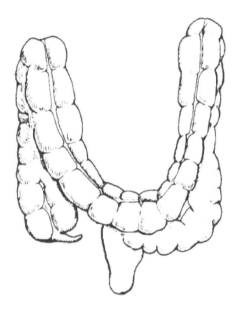

Enlarged Redundant Bowel

Chapter 3

Health Problems helped by Magnesium - D to I

Depression

At a time when advances in medical science and a growing use of natural remedies are reducing the frequency and severity of many diseases, depression appears to be heading in the opposite direction. Could that be due in part to the growing numbers of people who are deficient in magnesium?

Depression affects men and women of all ages, as well as children and teenagers, and is the world's most common mood disorder. And though depression is sometimes mistaken for the normal and temporary feelings of sadness and self-reproach that come with the everyday ups and downs of life, it is truly much more than that. Depression can be relatively minor, but it can also be a major, life-threatening illness. Rather than get into the rather lengthy criteria that are used to diagnose depression (these criteria are available from your doctor or easily found in the library or on the Internet), let me emphasise instead that depression is always treatable. Mild to moderate depression can often be treated effectively with supplements of fish oil, magnesium, tyrosine powder, B vitamins and the herb hypericum.

More severe and persistent clinical depression is very effectively alleviated with the modern generation of antidepressant drugs known as Selective Serotonin Reuptake Inhibitors (SSRIs). The SSRI antidepressant drugs can safely be taken along with a magnesium supplement.

Research dating back 80 or more years points to magnesium

as being one of the most effective components of a successful depression treatment plan, either taken alone, taken in conjunction with counselling, or taken along with counselling and prescribed medications. For instance, serotonins are the chemicals in the brain that promote contentment and cheerfulness – and magnesium is a very crucial factor in serotonin production. Case histories are available that show rapid recovery (a week or less) from mild to moderate depression if a magnesium supplement is taken with each meal and at bedtime. It has even been recommended that further study is needed into the possibility that magnesium deficiency is a component of most major depressive illnesses – and this is a recommendation that certainly has my support.

My book, "Help for Depression and Anxiety" provides a holistic plan for a happy and healthy nervous system. It discusses the use of the powerful amino acid, Tyrosine, to increase levels of the happy brain chemical Dopamine.

Diabetes and Syndrome X

Diabetes is a disease we're all familiar with. But do you know exactly what causes it? Well, to simplify it a bit … when you eat carbohydrates they are converted to glucose, a sugar your body uses for energy. Insulin is a hormone produced by your pancreas to control the amount of glucose in your blood. Without insulin, too much sugar stays in your blood.

There are two types of diabetes:

Type 1 diabetes occurs when your pancreas makes little or no insulin, and is a hereditary or autoimmune condition. It usually comes on early in life. Type 1 diabetes is also known as insulin dependent diabetes.

Type 2 diabetes occurs when your body produces enough insulin, but the insulin does not work efficiently in controlling blood sugar levels. It usually shows up later in life, and is often called adult-onset diabetes.

But regardless of the type, diabetes can cause serious problems with your blood vessels, heart, eyes, kidneys, legs and feet. As an example, it's estimated that two-thirds of all diabetics die from some type of heart disease.

Syndrome X is a precursor to diabetes type 2 and is caused by insulin resistance; this means that the body does not respond to insulin. To compensate, the pancreas makes more and more insulin – which eventually leads to excess levels of insulin in the blood. Insulin is a fat-storing hormone and this is why the vast majority of people with Syndrome X are overweight, especially in the abdominal area.

If you want to avoid adult-onset diabetes and/or Syndrome X, the wisest things you can do are to eat a low carbohydrate diet and make sure you are getting an adequate amount of magnesium. A low carbohydrate eating plan that gets your insulin and blood sugar levels down and promotes weight loss can be found in my book *Can't Lose Weight? Unlock the Secrets that KEEP you FAT.*

In my mind, there is more than ample evidence that diabetics need supplemental magnesium. For one thing, magnesium deficiency is extremely common in people with diabetes, and for another, we've already established that *(1)* heart problems kill the majority of diabetics and *(2)* that magnesium is essential to maintaining a healthy heart. Where Syndrome X is concerned, researchers have found that low magnesium levels are directly related to (a) muscle and fat cells becoming resistant to insulin and (b) pancreatic cells overproducing and secreting too much insulin.

Still, and in spite of the facts, you'll find a few reputable scientists who will tell you there is little evidence supporting routine magnesium supplementation for diabetics. I can only assume they've not done much research, or given the subject much thought, because the evidence is there; a low level of magnesium raises your risk for diabetes.

Eclampsia (Toxemia of Pregnancy)

Eclampsia, which is also known as Toxemia of pregnancy, refers to the coma and convulsive seizures that occur in small numbers of women in the third trimester of pregnancy or within the first 48 hours following delivery.

Eclampsia usually follows pre-eclampsia. Pre-eclampsia is a condition characterized by the new onset of high blood pressure (more than 140/90 millimeters of mercury) after 20 weeks of pregnancy.

Pre-eclampsia may progress rapidly from mild to severe and, if left untreated, to eclampsia. Eclampsia, if not treated, can be fatal.

Approximately 5 percent of pregnancies are complicated by pre-eclampsia. Of these patients, between 0.5 percent and 2 percent progress to eclampsia. The incidence is increased in women of low socio-economic status and extremes of age, and both pre-eclampsia and eclampsia account for significant worldwide death rates in pregnant women and new mothers and their infants.

The good news is that magnesium has been proven to be very effective in treating pregnancy-induced high blood pressure, and even the convulsions caused by eclampsia.

According to one report I read, magnesium was first used 100 years ago – in the early 1900s – to help prevent the seizures associated with eclampsia. In the years since, a number of studies have confirmed the wisdom of this early usage.

The Collaborative Eclampsia Trial matched magnesium sulphate against diazepam, an anti-anxiety and sedative drug, and phenytoin, an anticonvulsant drug, in a randomized study of nearly 1,700 women in a total of 10 countries. In both cases, magnesium proved superior. An even larger study, run from England, compared IV infusions of magnesium with infusions of a placebo in more than 10,000 women, to determine if magnesium could prevent the development of severe hypertension and convulsions. The women who received magnesium saw their chances of developing eclampsia reduced by 58 percent – a substantial improvement.

As a doctor who has done a lot of obstetrics, I'm very familiar with the many conditions that can complicate a pregnancy. It's reassuring to know that a mineral as safe and as easily available as magnesium can improve your chances of having a successful pregnancy.

Fibromyalgia

Fibromyalgia causes chronic muscle, connective tissue and soft tissue pain and tenderness that can occur anywhere in the body. Fibromyalgia won't permanently damage your body or destroy your joints – but the pain is often so severe that it may very well interfere with your day-to-day activities. Other possible associated symptoms are fatigue, headaches, stiffness, poor sleep and burning or tingling sensations.

Fibromyalgia can have several causes, though the end result is inflammation and spasm in the muscles and ligaments. The conventional approach is to treat this with exercise, physiotherapy, massage and anti-inflammatory drugs. There is a lot of evidence that the use of natural anti-inflammatory nutrients can control the symptoms. A good program would include fish oil, bone and joint nutrients (e.g. calcium, manganese, copper, boron and silica). Vitamin D3 is essential and you should have a blood test to check your Vitamin D level. Required doses of Vitamin D3 range from 1,000 to 10,000 units daily.

Natural bio-identical hormones such as Testosterone, Pregnenolone and/or DHEA can provide remarkable relief in men and women. For more information, call my Health Advisory Service in Australia on 02 4655 8855. In the USA phone 623 334 3232. Alternatively email ehelp@liverdoctor.com

Supplemental magnesium is essential for those with fibromyalgia. Magnesium can relieve much of the muscle tension and pain associated with the disorder, which is not surprising because of its ability to relax stiff and contracted muscles. Low magnesium levels are commonly found in fibromyalgia patients.

Turkish researchers recently determined that magnesium is one of the best and most effective treatment options for people with fibromyalgia. A similar study in the United States confirms that magnesium provides the "best evidence" for being effective in combating fibromyalgia. And when a group of fibromyalgia patients were treated with daily doses of magnesium for six weeks, their average level of pain – as measured on a tenderness scale – was reduced by two-thirds. Two weeks after some of the patients were switched to a placebo, their pain level had risen to the highest point ever. If pain and tenderness describe your problem, magnesium may be the solution.

Glaucoma

Glaucoma is the eye disease caused when the optic nerve at the back of the eye is damaged by increased pressure within the eye. This increased pressure (called elevated intraocular pressure) is the result of a build-up of fluid in the eye. Glaucoma is a major cause of blindness in adults and it is estimated that roughly two percent of the population over the age of 40 has glaucoma, with that number rising to 10 percent by age 70.

The most common glaucoma symptoms are a throbbing pain in the eye and blurred vision, but since not everyone has symptoms, it's recommended that once you reach the age of 45 you have an annual eye checkup, which includes a test of your eye pressure.

Overall, I've found there is a relative lack of research into the relationship between magnesium and glaucoma – as compared to magnesium and some of the other disorders we'll discuss. Still, there is enough information available through various sources to convince me that glaucoma patients may derive significant benefits from eating magnesium-rich foods and taking a daily supplement. In one study, for instance, 10 glaucoma patients were given 121.5 milligrams of magnesium twice a day for a month. At the end of that time frame, the patients reported improved vision.

Another study, one that focused on different nutrients and how they might improve the vision of glaucoma patients, found that magnesium does provide "potential benefit."

While I would certainly encourage additional research into the effects of magnesium on glaucoma, I can still say without reservation that making sure you get an adequate amount of magnesium would be a vital strategy for everyone who has the disorder.

Glaucoma sufferers should also increase their antioxidant intake via raw vegetable juicing and make sure that they eat yellow, orange, red and green fruits and vegetables. Also, take an antioxidant tablet containing selenium, zinc, vitamin E and vitamin C every day. Fish oil is also essential.

Avoid excess coffee and sugar, as these things will increase pressure within the eye (intraocular pressure).

Heart Attack

There is a very large and a very convincing body of evidence pointing to the key role magnesium plays in the overall health of your heart. Much of this evidence has been around for years – and has been largely ignored by many mainstream drug companies and doctors. That's slowly changing, however, and today more and more doctors and researchers are finding truth in the long-held minority belief that a magnesium deficiency may actually be responsible for many heart-related problems. Foremost among those problems is an acute myocardial infarction (AMI), which is doctor-speak for a heart attack.

Though entire books have been written on heart attacks, the simple explanation is that a heart attack is the result of complete or critical blockage of the blood flow to a part of the heart muscle. This normally occurs when a blood clot forms in one of the blood vessels (coronary arteries) that supply the heart muscle. When this happens the affected part of the heart muscle is severely damaged, often irreversibly so. It's a well-established fact that people who die of sudden heart attacks, or sudden severe heart arrythmias, will usually have a lower magnesium level than people of the same age who do not suffer with cadio-vascular disease.

Here are several facts about the role of magnesium in maintaining a healthy heart:

(1) The heart is the hardest-working muscle in your body and contains more magnesium than any of your other muscles

(2) Magnesium helps coordinate the activity of the heart muscle and regulates the rhythm of the heart beat

(3) Magnesium relaxes the coronary arteries to allow improved blood and oxygen delivery to the heart muscle

(4) Magnesium can thin the blood and thereby help prevent the formation of blood clots.

In addition, a number of studies in recent years have demonstrated that if you receive magnesium intravenously during the first hour you are hospitalized for an acute heart attack, your chances of survival will improve and there will be less likelihood of immediate and long-term complications. But to be completely fair on this subject, it has also been reported that one major trial found no significant reduction in the five-week mortality rate for patients who were treated with magnesium within 24 hours of their heart attack. These conflicting results have undoubtedly created some controversy within the medical community – but I and many other doctors stand firm in the belief that magnesium is absolutely essential for a healthy heart. And that's both before and after a heart attack.

In particular, magnesium should reduce the risk of sudden death from coronary artery spasm, severe sudden arrhythmia and reduced coronary artery flow.

The best way to use magnesium is as a preventative to reduce your risk of heart attack and/or sudden cardiac death.

High Blood Pressure

A number of studies in recent years have looked at the relationship between low magnesium levels and high blood pressure – with the majority of the evidence indicating that magnesium can and does significantly reduce blood pressure in many people. Not all studies have reached this conclusion, however, and some of the positive studies have been criticized as being flawed. As a result, I'd hope that research continues in this area, and that all future studies are carefully designed and controlled so that there can be no disputing the results.

Meanwhile, my own clinical experiences have been very positive and I have found that my hypertensive patients always get significant reductions, and sometimes large reductions, in their blood pressure. In mild to moderate elevations of blood pressure, a regular magnesium supplement along with regular exercise and weight loss usually restores a normal, healthy blood pressure.

Magnesium can also be taken along with blood pressure medication with no negative interactions; however, let your doctor know before you start taking it.

Blood pressure is the measurement of the force of blood flow against your artery walls as the heart beats. The top number records the systolic pressure, or the force that blood flow exerts on the artery walls as the heart contracts. The lower number, the diastolic pressure, is the force blood flow exerts on the artery walls when the heart is at rest, between heartbeats. If your blood pressure readings are consistently above 140 over 90 (140/90), you have high blood pressure, also known as hypertension. High blood pressure puts you at increased risk for a heart attack, a stroke, or kidney or eye damage and is a silent killer.

In my opinion, as well as in the opinion of many holistic doctors, magnesium can reduce elevated blood pressure by relaxing the muscles in the walls of your arteries, thereby allowing your blood to flow more freely.

In a study of 91 middle-aged and elderly women with mild to moderate high blood pressure who were not on medication, taking 480 mg of magnesium every day for six months resulted in blood pressure readings that were near normal.

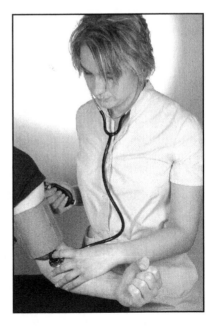

Another study that looked at dietary approaches to lowering blood pressure found that greater magnesium intake was definitely associated with a lower risk of high blood pressure. And to quote, "The evidence is strong enough that the Joint National Committee on Prevention, Detection, Evaluation and Treatment of High Blood Pressure recommends maintaining an adequate magnesium intake as a positive lifestyle modification for preventing and managing high blood pressure."

Insomnia

As I started my research into the link between magnesium levels and insomnia, I was disappointed to find very little literature on the subject. While I did turn up a couple of articles, they didn't concentrate on insomnia per se. Rather, they were on the use of magnesium as therapy for periodic limb movements during sleep (PLMS) and restless leg syndrome (RLS), two conditions known to contribute to sleep disturbances and insomnia. Magnesium is thought to be useful in treating both PLMS and RLS, which I certainly consider good news. It is also something I have found to be true with my own patients. And after all, treating the conditions that cause a disorder is better than just alleviating the symptoms, right? I would definitely say so – and in this thought I emphasise the importance of magnesium to people who have problems sleeping.

Insomnia is generally defined as "having difficulty falling asleep" or "frequent or early awakening." The three most common causes of insomnia are -

(1) depression

(2) anxiety

(3) stress (or tension)

Guess what? Magnesium is a reliable remedy for all three.

We've already touched on how magnesium can help pull you from the depths of depression, as well as help relieve the angst that accompanies anxiety. In just a bit, we'll be looking at the important role magnesium plays in the reduction of stress. So, if this miracle mineral can eliminate – or at the very least, reduce – the three main causes of insomnia, it only follows that increasing magnesium intake should work wonders for people who are magnesium deficient and have trouble sleeping.

More research into the subject would certainly be welcome, but as far as I'm concerned there is already ample evidence to recommend magnesium as a remedy for almost everyone who has difficulty sleeping. I also recommend my book titled **Tired of not Sleeping? – Holistic remedies for a good night's sleep**, as it contains extensive help for anyone with sleep problems.

Irritability

Irritability, which is defined in one of my medical dictionaries as "a quick response to annoyance; impatience", appears to me to be increasingly common in today's world. You see it everywhere – from the workplace to the supermarket, in traffic and at public events.

You also see it in people of all ages. Children can be just as irritable as their grandparents, parents are certainly not exempt, and working people seem particularly susceptible. Part of the blame, I suspect, lies with the fast pace of our lives and the daily pressure to succeed that many of us feel. Magnesium deficiency is quite likely another significant cause.

Though there has been very little research to date on how low levels of magnesium might lead specifically to irritability, there are a lot of related studies – studies into the origins of anxiety, chronic depression and panic disorders, for instance. These and several other related conditions all have irritability as a symptom, and all may be improved or prevented by increasing your daily intake of magnesium.

In a study of suicide statistics (suicide can be the end result of severe depression), a French scientist found that "those who regularly absorbed a good amount of magnesium salts have a more stable equilibrium, they support adversity with more calm and do not renounce everything to avoid some sorrow... The use of magnesium permits one to support adversity with more serenity".

I don't know about you, but I place a high value on serenity – both in myself and in my patients. If it can be provided by something as natural, as easily obtainable and as non-habit forming as magnesium, that alone is reason enough to make sure you are never again magnesium deficient.

Chapter 4

Health Problems helped by Magnesium - K – S

Kidney Stones

Most any doctor who has practised general medicine will likely tell you that kidney stones are one of the most common and most painful, patient complaints. It is estimated that perhaps 10 percent of all adult males will experience a kidney stone during their lifetimes – and it is an experience most will never forget. One victim who has been quoted in print said the pain of passing a kidney stone is comparable to "passing broken bottles, old razor blades, molten lead and sulfuric acid garnished with bits of rusty barbed wire". Ouch!

Kidney stones form from minerals in the urine, with approximately 80 percent of all stones composed of calcium salts. There are also a number of metabolic diseases, such as gout, that can cause kidney stones to develop, though the most common cause – not drinking enough water – is also the most easily remedied. At the same time, anyone who has a history of kidney stones should make sure that he (males are affected more often than females) or she is getting adequate amounts of magnesium, as magnesium is known to prevent the formation of kidney stones.

In one study, 56 subjects with a kidney stone history were given 200 milligrams of magnesium twice a day for two years. On average, the number of kidney stones they developed was reduced by more than 50 percent. Another study showed that a magnesium-deficient diet is one of the quickest ways to cause kidney stones in rats (maybe that explains the mysterious moans some people hear coming from inside their walls late at night!), while still another study found that patients with a history of kidney stones became stone-free after taking magnesium tablets for "only a very short time." And there are several reports of kidney stone patients who passed no stones while taking magnesium, only to have their stones return once they discontinued their magnesium therapy.

As well as taking a magnesium supplement, I always advise my patients with kidney stones to make a raw juice to reduce the acidity of their blood and urine – you need to juice celery, mint, cucumber, carrot, ginger and apples. Also make sure you drink at least two liters of water daily and cut back on alcohol.

Even if I weren't a doctor it would be apparent that when it comes to kidney stones, magnesium can indeed work miracles.

Migraine Headaches

Migraine headaches – perhaps the most painful of all headaches – are caused by excessive constriction (narrowing) and then excessive dilation (expansion) of the blood vessels in your head. This explains why migraine sufferers complain of a severe pulsating or throbbing pain in the head. Migraines are surprisingly common, affecting an estimated 20 percent of all men and 25 percent to 30 percent of all women at some point in their lives. That's a lot of people, hundreds of millions in fact, so it should help a lot of you breathe easier to know that you can count on magnesium for at least some relief.

Several different studies have determined that a magnesium deficiency can set the stage for a migraine, with one researcher saying, "The importance of magnesium deficiency in the development of migraine headaches is clearly established... The available evidence suggests that up to 50 percent of patients during an acute migraine attack have lowered levels of ... magnesium. Infusion of magnesium results in a rapid and sustained relief of an acute migraine in such patients".

According to other reports, magnesium can lessen the severity of a migraine by reducing the constrictions and spasms in the arteries that cause them in the first place. This improves and stabilizes the circulation of blood to the head area, including the brain.

In a double-blind study of 81 people with a history of recurrent migraines, some of the patients were given oral magnesium daily while the others received a placebo. By the ninth week, nearly 42 percent of the magnesium group reported a reduction in the frequency of their attacks, as opposed to only 15.8 percent of patients in the placebo group. But again, to be perfectly fair, I have seen results from a similar study that found magnesium, when compared to a placebo, provided no benefits in reducing the frequency of migraines.

My personal experience, along with the experiences of many of my colleagues, convinces me that this latter study was possibly flawed in some way, though I admit to having no hard evidence to support this belief. What I can and do support, however, is the opinion of the researcher who stated, "Because of an excellent safety profile and low cost, and despite the lack of definitive studies, we feel that a trial of oral magnesium supplementation can be recommended to a majority of migraine sufferers."

I have seen many of my patients reduce the frequency and severity of many types of headaches by taking 400 mg daily of elemental magnesium. This includes tension headaches, cluster headaches and migraines.

If the migraine headaches are usually associated with nausea and vomiting, it is also important to improve the function of the liver. This can be done by increasing the amount of raw salad vegetables and raw juices in the diet and by taking a good liver tonic – see *www.liverdoctor.com*

Fish oil supplements can also help to reduce the inflammatory component of headaches – take two capsules of 1000 mg each, twice daily just before food. The liquid form of fish oil is much more effective and doses vary from 1 teaspoon to 1 tablespoon twice daily, just before food.

All migraine sufferers should ensure a good intake of water with the aim of drinking two liters (2 quarts) daily. This will improve the circulation of blood to the brain. Dehydration will increase the frequency and severity of headaches.

Testimonial

Dear Dr Cabot:

I am writing to tell you about the great relief I have obtained from taking magnesium tablets. Since the age of 24, I have been suffering from severe migraines that would put me to bed for at least a day. They would often start with flashing lights and nausea and just a dull ache on one side of my head. Then the pain would get worse and turn into a pulsating throbbing pain all over my head. I could not move or stand the light. Sometimes these frightening headaches would awaken me in the early hours of the morning and I would be scared I was going to have a stroke!

I have tried many different drugs over the years but they had side effects and only relieved the pain for a few hours. I nearly became addicted to pain killing injections. Then I read about the beneficial effects that magnesium could have on migraines and I thought to myself – no, it's too simple, how could a natural substance help such severe pain?

However I was desperate; I thought, well I have nothing to lose. I started taking two Magnesium Complete tablets twice daily and found that gradually my headaches became less frequent, and when I got one, it was not as bad. I have not had a migraine for five months now and I can't believe my luck!

My life has changed in such a great way and I no longer worry about having to cancel things and miss out on the things I love to do. I would also like to thank you for your book on raw juicing, as I am sure that the juice recipes I have been using have also helped to prevent the headaches. I no longer feel nauseated or have to live on painkillers and I think that something must have helped my liver – perhaps the magnesium or perhaps the raw juices.

Julia Mac Donald
Brisbane, Queensland

Mitral Valve Prolapse

The sound that most of us associate with a beating heart is the sound of heart valves closing as they regulate the direction of blood flow in the heart. But in the 5 percent of the population that's affected with the condition called mitral valve prolapse, there's an additional sound caused when the valve between the two left chambers of the heart billows abnormally when the lower chamber contracts. It's a sound that has been described as similar to a "parachute being snapped in the wind." And when the valve does not seal properly, blood may leak backwards to cause a heart murmur.

Although heart specialists will generally tell you that mitral valve prolapse is hereditary and won't cause life-threatening problems in most cases, it can still create symptoms that range from fatigue and shortness of breath to chest pain, heart palpitations, dizziness and anxiety. The anxiety, in particular, is understandable, because who wants to go around worrying about having a defective heart valve?

Fortunately, there is a substantial body of research that has found a link between low levels of magnesium and mitral valve prolapse symptoms. According to reports I've read, an estimated 85 percent of all people with mitral valve prolapse have chronic magnesium deficiency.

It's extremely important to note, however, that while magnesium can relieve your symptoms, and according to some studies may even be able to improve mitral valve prolapse, magnesium should not be considered a cure, nor should it replace professional medical care and attention.

I do not want to mislead you here, so this is worth repeating. If you have been diagnosed with mitral valve prolapse, magnesium may

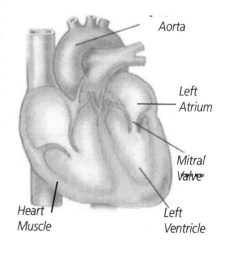

Aorta

Left Atrium

Mitral Valve

Heart Muscle

Left Ventricle

relieve many of your symptoms. But magnesium cannot cure you. Please be clear on this and do not expect more from magnesium than it can realistically provide.

Multiple Sclerosis

Multiple sclerosis, or MS as it is commonly known, is a disease I particularly dislike because it tends to occur early in life, with about 65 percent to 70 percent of all cases affecting young women and men between the ages of 20 and 40. Statistics show that onset is rarely after age 50. It is also an insidious disease – one that may progress steadily in some patients, while other patients will experience acute attacks followed by partial or complete temporary remission of symptoms. And though the actual cause of MS has never been conclusively identified, we do know that the gradual loss of the insulating sheath (myelin sheath) that surrounds nerves leads to the progressive nerve disturbances that characterise MS. The prevailing theory is that the body's autoimmune process is abnormally activated to attack the myelin sheaths.

MS damages the central nervous system and because of this, signs of MS-related nerve dysfunction can appear in many different locations throughout the body. Typical symptoms of MS include muscle weakness, paralysis of limbs, blurred vision or loss of vision, dizziness, tingling sensations, numbness, fatigue and tremors, with clumsiness and muscle contractions that cause stiff and awkward movements (spasticity) also being common.

The value of magnesium in relation to multiple sclerosis is two-fold:

1. Magnesium is usually depressed in the central nervous system tissues of MS patients, so keeping your magnesium levels high might possibly serve as a preventative measure and reduce your risk of getting the disease. Experimental and clinical studies have found that magnesium affects the maintenance and function of nerve cells, and that a magnesium deficit could very well be a risk factor in the development of MS.

2. Magnesium may significantly reduce many of the symptoms of MS. For example, magnesium is known to help muscles

relax, reduce tremors, reduce spasticity and increase energy levels – all of which would definitely improve the wellbeing of most MS patients. Magnesium also helps produce cellular energy and is needed for nerve impulse transmission.

One medical report I read stated, "It is highly regrettable that the deficiency of such an inexpensive, low-toxicity nutrient (as magnesium) results in diseases that cause incalculable suffering and expense throughout the world." I couldn't agree more – and would only add that multiple sclerosis is definitely one of those diseases.

MS sufferers may also find that the progression of their disease can be greatly slowed down by taking regular supplements of selenium, vitamins C and E and D, and fish oil.

MS sufferers must avoid Vitamin D deficiency and should have a blood test from their doctor to check their serum Vitamin D levels. Vitamin D deficiency will increase the severity of MS.

In some female MS patients with menstrual problems and after childbirth, the use of natural progesterone cream in a dose of 50 to 100 mg daily can provide a substantial improvement in MS symptoms.

Muscle Cramps

A muscle cramp is a relatively simple disorder caused by the involuntary, and the usually brief, contraction of a muscle. Though they're more uncomfortable than they are dangerous, unless you happen to get one, say, when you are swimming, muscle cramps can still be very painful. Muscle cramps can also be very distressing if they occur during competitive sports or at night, when they awaken you from a deep sleep.

Imbalances in certain minerals known as electrolytes – magnesium being one – are linked to muscle cramps and spasms. A lot of people are undoubtedly familiar with the term "electrolyte" from sports drink advertisements. But if you don't know the particulars, an electrolyte is an ionized salt in the body's cells, with these salts including calcium, potassium and magnesium. For a muscle to do its job and function properly, you must have a proper level of all three of these salts, and here's where the problem with cramps starts. While most of us generally have adequate amounts of calcium and potassium, the same is not true of magnesium – yet magnesium has been called the key that unlocks muscle cells and lets in the calcium and potassium so they can do their jobs. Without the key – without the magnesium – your muscles may be in less than perfect health. Hence, muscle cramps.

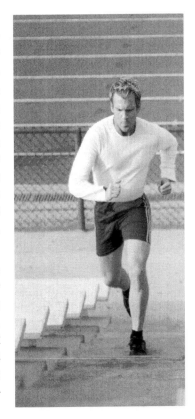

There is little doubt that a strong case can be made for the importance of magnesium in preventing muscle cramps. There are studies, in fact, that show magnesium reduces leg cramp distress in both pregnant women and in "non-pregnant" individuals.

Some people may find that increasing their magnesium intake relieves cramping almost immediately, while others may need a month or more to reverse a long-standing deficiency and see any results. Either way, the sooner you increase your magnesium levels, the sooner your muscle cramps will retreat and become a distant memory.

Testimonial - This true story will give you a laugh!

Dear Dr Sandra Cabot,

I have been taking magnesium for many years ever since I discovered that it cured my terrible night cramps. I don't think there is anything more debilitating than a sudden attack of cramping muscles. I had been a sufferer for too long and also had twitching eyelids, cramped fingers and toes, but the worse thing was the cramps in my calves and feet that would suddenly grab me whilst sleeping. The latter were absolute agony that woke me up gasping in pain; they would last 20 minutes to an hour, forcing me to hop around the bedroom crying for help. This would usually awaken my husband, who was also a victim of cramps, so sometimes there would be two of us hopping around the bedroom and we could see the funny side of it – but not often.

We became desperate and tried all the folk remedies and old wives' tales for relief. One of these included putting a lump of camphor in an old sock, which we left in the bottom of the bed in between the sheets. Phew, it stunk; we would get into bed and felt as though we were in the old folk's home! But we were desperate enough to try anything! All to no avail – until a friend who was one of your patients told me about ultra potent magnesium powder. I rushed out to the health food store and bought some and thank God, this produced the greatest, most wonderful change in our lives. All my symptoms were cured within two weeks and my husband found relief after three weeks. My husband also found that the magnesium cured his painful muscle spasms that occurred in his rectum, and this relieved a very embarrassing problem for him. We could not believe the huge difference that magnesium made in our lives and our sleep – we are never without magnesium in our house or when we are away travelling.

Jacqueline Wise

Perth WA

Muscle Weakness

We've already established that magnesium is beneficial for muscles, increases your energy level and helps relieve tension (tension can certainly cause muscles to become overtired). Muscle weakness is yet another one of those conditions that are rarely if ever treated as a separate disorder by researchers studying magnesium; rather, muscle weakness is just included as a symptom of other disorders.

But no matter how you choose to define it, muscle weakness can still be very debilitating – and it will usually respond to magnesium supplementation. A medical paper written in Japan described how a patient with chronic fatigue syndrome had suffered with muscle weakness (along with other symptoms) for years. Nothing at all, including a number of prescription medications, seemed to help her condition, until she was administered magnesium for six weeks. Her muscle weakness improved, and after more than a year in the hospital she was able to leave. A U.S. study that took place in a hospital ICU (intensive care unit) found that a deficiency in magnesium can lead to respiratory muscle weakness. Still another study, this one on normal and abnormal muscle function, determined that low levels of magnesium are associated with muscle weakness.

Unfortunately, however, research studies that look at the relationship between magnesium and muscle weakness as a stand-alone disorder are still relatively few and far between. And this will likely remain the case until more researchers and scientists wake up to the wonderful and amazing healing power of magnesium. Meanwhile, I truly hope that this lack of information doesn't prevent or discourage anyone with a muscle problem from considering magnesium as a potential solution. It may just be the best option of all.

Parkinson's Disease

Parkinson's disease, which rarely affects anyone under the age of 50, occurs when the brain cells that produce a chemical called dopamine don't work properly. Dopamine is necessary to control muscle movement, so symptoms of Parkinson's disease will usually include stiff muscles, slow movements, shuffling gait, poor coordination, clumsiness, balance problems, and tremors in the hands, arms and/or legs.

There is no known treatment guaranteed to stop or reverse the breakdown of brain cells that causes Parkinson's disease – but medical research has uncovered two important facts:

1. Most Parkinson's disease patients have confirmed low magnesium levels in multiple areas of their brain.

2. A magnesium deficiency can and often does contribute to substantial muscle weakness and tremor.

One of the interesting – and at times, frustrating – aspects of researching the benefits of magnesium is that you frequently have to dig very deep to find study results, in large part because so many supposedly intelligent scientists tend to either ignore or discount the tremendous importance of magnesium to your overall health.

In digging into the relationship between magnesium and Parkinson's disease, I turned up a review of a study done in Hungary, in which three researchers looked at how plants take aluminium from the soil and are poisoned as a result. The study found that if farmers use fertilizers containing magnesium, this inhibits or decreases aluminium concentrations in the soil. What does this have to do with Parkinson's disease? Well, at the end of the review it was noted that "aluminium may be implicated in Parkinson's disease," and since magnesium moderates the effect of this "toxic element" in plants, it may do the same "in the human organism" as well.

Is this statement accurate? That's hard to answer either way with certainty. But since we do know that many Parkinson's disease victims are magnesium deficient, and since it has been proven that magnesium is good for the muscles, it doesn't take a degree in science to figure magnesium might either help prevent the disease, or help relieve its symptoms, or both.

As well as taking magnesium, patients with Parkinson's disease can be helped by supplements of selenium, vitamins C and E and D, and fish oil. Raw juicing of vegetables and fruits can also help to reduce the brain inflammation associated with Parkinson's disease.

The regular use of large amounts of the artificial sweetener aspartame has been associated with an increased risk and/or premature onset of Parkinson's disease.

See www.dorway.com

Stress

If you say the word "stress" most people will automatically think of such things as pressure to excel at work, a family fight, financial hardship, working excess hours, getting stuck in traffic, etc. In reality, stress is much more complex, covering everything from the physical (athletic exertion to surgery and pregnancy), to the emotional (anxiety to depression and anger), to the environmental (industrial pollution, noise and passive cigarette smoke). It has even been said – and I certainly agree – that a magnesium deficiency is a stress in its own right ... and if you are one of those people who are chronically stressed you can quickly become magnesium deficient, even if you regularly eat all of the right foods.

To try and simplify what is actually a very complex process, let me just say that exposure to stress can increase the level of adrenaline, a stress hormone, in your blood. As this occurs, magnesium is released from your cells into the blood stream – to be used in energy production, to help your heart, and to increase muscle function – before eventually being eliminated in the urine. It follows, then, that over time stress tends to deplete the magnesium in our bodies. This becomes an even bigger problem if we are magnesium deficient to begin with. Now, add to this the fact that a low magnesium level causes us to be more sensitive to stress in the first place, and you can see how easy it would be to get into a vicious cycle of stress lowering our magnesium levels, which makes us more receptive to stress, which lowers our magnesium even more, which makes us even more receptive to stress, etc., etc. This could eventually lead to a stress breakdown of the mind and body.

Magnesium could be the circuit breaker that protects your central nervous system from dangerous overload. That's why I call magnesium "the great relaxer."

Unfortunately, the situation can get even worse because the magnesium depletion caused by stress can then open the body's door to everything from a migraine headache and high blood pressure to insomnia, glaucoma and a heart attack.

So the bottom line here is that how we respond to the various stressors in our lives – both those we recognise and those we don't – goes a long way toward determining quality and quantity of life and how healthy we are.

I'd be the first to say that no one can live without experiencing some degree of stress from time to time. It's just impossible.

Even if you live in one of the world's most remote and beautiful areas and have very little contact with other people, there are still going to be those days when the local insects get into your dwindling sugar supply or your roof develops a major leak during the middle of the rainy season.

It's imperative that you try to recognise what's causing the stress in your life, and then manage and reduce it as much as possible through changing your lifestyle, practising relaxation techniques, getting adequate exercise, eating a healthy diet, and so on. And always remember the importance of magnesium – which along with its other title of "the great relaxer" has definitely shown promise as "the great stress buster."

Stroke

A stroke causes damage to the brain by interrupting its blood supply, usually when a blood clot forms inside an artery or an artery actually bursts.

Within a few minutes, the nerve cells in the brain are starved for oxygen, become damaged, and can die. If you survive, remaining symptoms can include impaired vision and speech, changed behavior, loss of thought processes and memory, or the inability to move different parts of your body. The exact effects will vary greatly from person to person, depending on which brain cells are damaged, how much of the brain is affected, and how quickly blood resumes flowing to the affected area.

Magnesium offers hope to both "potential" and "actual" stroke victims on a couple of fronts. To begin, one way you can help prevent a stroke is to control one or more of the risk factors for stroke. The leading risk factors are high blood pressure, heart disease, smoking, dehydration, diabetes and other disorders that can negatively affect your blood vessels. As we've already pointed out, magnesium is known to have a positive impact on each of these conditions, so it naturally follows that magnesium will be beneficial in reducing or perhaps altogether eliminating the likelihood of you having a stroke.

But in the event that a stroke does occur, magnesium can also help with your recovery – as long as it is quickly administered.

In one study, 20 patients who were identified by the responding paramedics as having had an acute stroke were given intravenous magnesium sulphate within one hour of being afflicted, followed by additional magnesium infusions over the next 24 hours. It was reported that 25 percent of these patients experienced a "dramatic recovery."

Another case study, this one reported in a review of the use of magnesium to treat arterial disease over a period of 34 years, involved a 57-year-old woman who "had a gradual onset of marked weakness and loss of sensation in her left arm, hand, leg and foot that failed to improve during three months of standard treatment." She was then given an injection of magnesium, which caused her symptoms to disappear for 12 hours – though they came back. This was followed, however, by a course of injections that led to a full recovery.

Other case studies I've seen tell similar stories, and this leads me to believe two things: (1) magnesium does provide definite stroke-related benefits, both preventive and after the fact, and (2) the medical profession needs to do a lot more research in this area, as strokes are a leading cause of morbidity and mortality in our population.

Magnesium can help to control high blood pressure, which is the leading cause of stroke. Magnesium helps to open up the arteries to the brain and optimize blood flow to critical areas of the brain. Anyone with high blood pressure who is serious about reducing his or her risk of stroke should be taking a daily magnesium supplement.

I would also encourage people at risk of stroke, and that's a huge percentage of the population, to boost their intake of vitamin C by taking a regular vitamin C supplement and increasing their intake of fresh citrus fruits, berries and capsicums. Vitamin C deficiency is very common, and is a significant risk factor for strokes, both thrombotic and hemorrhagic in origin.

Another way to greatly reduce your risk of strokes is to eat oily fish (such as sardines, herring, salmon and tuna) and/or take fish oil liquid or capsules.

Sudden Infant Death Syndrome

Sudden Infant Death Syndrome, or SIDS as it's more commonly known these days, is not only last on this list, it is also the final link in what I hope you now see is an interconnected chain of disorders and symptoms, that affect all parts of the body yet still have one thing in common; they can all be improved or prevented with the proper dosage of magnesium.

SIDS, sometimes called "crib death," is defined as "the sudden death of an infant younger than one year of age that remains unexplained after a thorough investigation, including a complete autopsy, examination of the death scene, and review of the clinical history. It is a diagnosis of exclusion in that there are no specific autopsy findings to account for the death."

In previous chapters, I've mentioned several times that magnesium is good for your muscles. In a review of 19 case-controlled studies that looked at the relationship between SIDS and babies sleeping on their stomachs, researchers found an overall higher rate of SIDS in infants who usually slept in this position.

The original studies were conducted in Australia, New Zealand, England, France and the Netherlands, and the results first led to changes in the sleeping positions of babies, and then to declines of 50 percent or more in the SIDS rate. As to what this has to do with muscles and magnesium, two additional studies showed that babies sleeping face down could be in jeopardy if they lacked the muscle strength to change positions or turn their heads to rescue themselves from a life-threatening position. There is data to support the theory that magnesium deficiency can at times be the cause of this muscle weakness – while an adequate intake of magnesium could rapidly reverse such weakness.

Children under the age of nine are best given a magnesium supplement in the form of a liquid or powder that can be dissolved in water or juice. Older children can be given a magnesium tablet. Breast feeding women need to eat plenty of foods high in magnesium (see page 67) and they and their infants will benefit greatly from the mother taking supplements of fish oil, iodine, Vitamin C, Vitamin D and magnesium whilst breast feeding; these nutrients will support the strength and growth of the muscles and nervous system.

Magnesium deficiency, which causes so many different problems in so many people of all ages, "is at least one unifying factor" that explains an increase of SIDS in infants who are prone to sleeping face down. Children with irritability, asthma, muscle spasms or hidden (sub clinical) epileptic fits, could have a higher risk of SIDS – thankfully magnesium can assist in all these problems.

Please, don't take chances with the life of your child by ignoring the possibility that he or she could be magnesium deficient.

Children are often picky eaters and it can be difficult to get them to eat enough foods that are high in magnesium - see page 67 for a list of foods high in magnesium. Symptoms of magnesium deficiency in children can include irritability, anxiety, headaches, muscle cramps, bed wetting, facial twitching, abdominal colic, wheezing, constipation and poor sleeping patterns.

Also don't forget to include a fish oil supplement (available in liquid form) whilst you are breast feeding, and/or give it to your infant, as omega 3 fatty acids are important in the brain's control of breathing and heart rate.

To Conclude

My list of the conditions that can be helped with magnesium covers the most common problems that are known to be associated with magnesium deficiency. I'm confident it could be expanded with further research, though my primary focus here has been to look at the magnesium-related disorders that affect the most people. I've also used these disorders to try and drive home the point that no part of your body truly functions on a stand-alone basis. Magnesium is a vital key that enables your cells to produce energy and communicate with other cells. This applies to cells found in the brain, the nerves, the heart and skeletal muscles, the smooth muscles in your arteries and intestines, and the hormonal glands.

Little wonder that your whole body will be affected adversely by a magnesium deficiency. This is why **Magnesium: The Miracle Mineral** is so important; it has been written to awaken you to the profound health benefits that can be achieved by ensuring that you are not deficient in magnesium.

The Chlorophyll Molecule

Mg = *Magnesium*

Magnesium is at the centre of the chlorophyll molecule

The chlorophyll molecule, which gives green color to plants, is rich in magnesium.

Those who do not eat green colored vegetables and fruits are likely to be magnesium deficient.

No wonder magnesium is the energy mineral for plants and humans!

Magnesium:
The Miracle Mineral

Chapter 5
Diet and Magnesium

If you held any doubts about the power of magnesium before you began reading Magnesium: The Miracle Mineral, I would hope that they have long since been dispelled and you are now ready to look at your eating habits, as well as those of your family, through magnesium-tinted glasses.

Taking a magnesium supplement can be a very good option, and depending on your personal circumstances it may even be the best option. It is also important to eat a diet rich in magnesium-laden foods. A wide variety of foods fall into this category – and the vast majority are not only tasty and generally easy to find, they often contain many other healthy nutrients as well.

It's important to realize that along with your current eating habits (be they good, bad or ugly), your age, your body weight, your sex and even the type of work you do can have an impact on how much magnesium you need to ingest on a daily basis.

Athletes who exercise strenuously can quickly become low in magnesium, as can both men and women who labour for a living, especially if they work outdoors in the sun. The reason: excessive perspiration and using the body's large muscle groups deplete magnesium. Also, new mothers who breast feed their babies require a higher magnesium intake, and as I've already noted, people older than 70 tend to both absorb less magnesium and excrete more in their urine.

A range of other lifestyle, environmental and medical circumstances – from emotional stress, alcohol abuse and diuretic use to gastrointestinal disease and the acid rain that washes magnesium from the soil – can likewise have a profound effect on your magnesium levels. As can everything from dieting to drinking too many soft drinks. Water that comes from wells, which oftentimes has naturally high levels of magnesium, may be subject to magnesium depletion if fluoride is added – a common practice in many communities.

Even how you cook your food can have an impact on your magnesium intake. If you boil leafy vegetables and then discard the water, some portion of the magnesium is also being discarded. (Tip: Instead of throwing this water away, save it and use it later when cooking rice or making soup.)

There are a number of other ways, too, in which your body's magnesium supply can be depleted, and for a refresher on this information I'd ask you to refer back to Chapter 1.

For most people, I'm sure the question now on your mind is exactly what can I eat to ensure a good supply of dietary magnesium? Well, to answer that question I've prepared the following chart to show you many of the foods with the highest magnesium content.

Each line in the chart will list a food, a common measure for that food, and the magnesium content of that measure in milligrams, with 100 milligrams (mg) being equal to 0.0035 of an ounce (oz). Please understand that the magnesium content is just an approximation – a close approximation but an approximation nonetheless.

You may well come upon similar charts that offer slightly different numbers, but many of the foods and figures in my chart were taken from the U. S. Department of Agriculture (USDA) Database for Standard Reference, which is as accurate or more accurate than what you'll find anywhere else.

Table of magnesium content of foods

Food	Measure	Milligrams (mg)
Almonds	24 nuts	78
Apricots, canned	1 cup	24
Artichokes	1 cup	101
Asparagus, boiled	1 cup	23
Avocado	1/2 cup	35
Bagel, plain	1 bagel	26
Baked beans, canned	1 cup	89
Bananas	1 cup	44
Bean & Ham soup, canned	1 cup	46
Beans, blacked boiled	1 cup	120
Beans, lima cooked	1/2 cup	63
Beetroot, boiled	1 cup	39
Bread crumbs	1 cup	46
Bread, whole wheat	1 slice	24
Broccoli, boiled	1 cup	37
Brussels sprouts, boiled	1 cup	37
Cashew nuts	28 grams	74
Cheese, ricotta	1 cup	37
Chestnuts	1 cup	47
Chicken & veg. soup, canned	1 cup	24
Chicken, grilled	1/2 breast	34
Chicken, stewed	1 cup	31
Chocolate bar	49 grams	42
Chocolate cake	1 piece	30
Cocoa powder	1 tablespoon	27
Coffee, brewed	60 mls (2oz)	48
Collard greens	1 cup	51
Cornmeal, yellow whole grain	1 cup	155
Crab, blue	84 grams	28
Cucumber, raw	1 large	34
Dates, dried	1 cup	62
Duck, roasted	1/2 duck	44
Fish, halibut	1/2 a fillet	170

Table of magnesium content

Food	Measure	Milligrams (mg)
Flour, buckwheat	1 cup	301
Flour, wheat	1 cup	166
Flour, white	1 cup	28
Grapefruit juice, frozen	1 can	79
Green pea soup, canned	1 cup	40
Green peas, frozen	1 cup	46
Green snap beans, frozen	1 cup	32
Hazelnuts	28 grams	46
Kale, boiled	1 cup	23
Kidney beans, canned	1/2 cup	35
Kiwi fruit	1 medium	23
Kohlrabi, boiled	1 cup	31
Lamb, braised	84 grams	25
Lentils, cooked	1/2 cup	35
Lettuce, iceberg	1 head	49
Lobster	84 grams	30
Macadamia nuts	10-12 nuts	33
Macaroni	1 cup	25
Milk condensed , canned	1 cup	80
Milk, chocolate	1 cup	53
Milk, evaporated	1 cup	60
Milk, full cream	1 cup	24
Milk, soy	1 cup	47
Minestrone soup, canned	1 cup	31
Miso sauce	1 cup	29
Nuts, mixed dry roasted	28 grams	64
Muffin, oat bran	1 muffin	89
Mushrooms, canned	1 cup	23
Oat bran	1 cup	221
Oatmeal, instant with water	1 cup	55
Orange juice, fresh	1 cup	27
Oysters, raw	6 medium	39
Parsnips, boiled	1 cup	45

Table of magnesium content

Food	Measure	Milligrams (mg)
Paw Paw	1 medium	30
Peanut butter	1 tablespoon	25
Peanuts, roasted	28 grams	50
Pears	1 pear	22
Peas, black eyed cooked	1/2 cup	43
Pecan pie	1 piece	32
Pecans	20 halves	34
Pine nuts, dried	28 grams	66
Pineapple, canned	1 cup	41
Pistachio nuts	28 grams	34
Pork loin	84 grams	27
Potato chips	28 grams	25
Potato, boiled	1 cup	31
Potato, mashed	1 cup	38
Potato, baked	1 potato	33
Potato, fried	1 large	66
Prawns, fried	6-8 prawns	39
Prunes, stewed	1 cup	50
Pumpkin seeds	28 grams	151
Raisins, seedless	1 cup	48
Raspberries, frozen	1 cup	33
Rhubarb	1 cup	29
Rice, brown	1 cup	84
Rice, white	1 cup	57
Rice, wild	1 cup	52
Salad with chicken	1 1/2 cups	33
Salmon	1/2 fillet	48
Sandwich, canned tuna	1 sandwich	79
Sandwich, chicken fillet	1 sandwich	35
Sandwich, roast beef	1 sandwich	67
Seeds, sesame	1 tablespoon	28
Sirloin, lean top	84 grams	27
Soybeans, boiled	1 cup	147

Table of magnesium content

Food	Measure	Milligrams (mg)
Spaghetti, whole wheat	1 cup	42
Spinach, boiled	1 cup	157
Spinach, canned	1 cup	163
Spinach, frozen	1 cup	131
Spinach, raw chopped, pressed	1 cup	110
Squash, boiled	1 cup	43
Sunflower seeds	1/4 cup	41
Sweet corn, canned	1 cup	48
Sweet corn, frozen	1 cup	31
Sweet potato, baked	1 potato	29
Tofu	1/4 block	37
Tomato paste	1 cup	134
Tomato puree	1 cup	60
Tomato sauce	1 cup	47
Tomato soup, canned	1 cup	22
Tomatoes, stewed	1 cup	31
Trout, rainbow	84 grams	27
Tuna salad	1 cup	39
Tuna, fresh	84 grams	54
Turkey, roasted	1 cup	36
Veal, braised	84 grams	25
Vegetable juice	1 cup	27
Vegetables, mixed	1 cup	40
Watermelon	1 wedge	31
Wheat bran	2 tablespoons	45
White beans, canned	1 cup	134
Yoghurt, plain	small container	43

Green vegetables, especially dark green leafy vegetables, such as spinach and broccoli, are excellent sources of magnesium because they contain the green pigment known as chlorophyll. The chlorophyll molecule is very rich in magnesium - see page 64. Remember Popeye the sailor man? Popeye was the cartoon character who boosted his strength with spinach!

You can see from my table that legumes (beans, peas and lentils), nuts and seeds and whole unrefined grains are also good sources. Refined grains are low in magnesium because when white flour is processed the magnesium rich germ and bran are removed. Choose breads made from whole grain flours instead of white processed breads.

Many herbs and spices contain large amounts of magnesium, such as - cilantro (coriander), dill, celery seed, sage, dried mustard, basil, parsley, fennel seed, cumin seed, tarragon, marjoram, poppy seed and curry powder.

Culinary seaweeds are very high in magnesium, as well as other immune boosting minerals, and I encourage you to include them in your diet. There are various culinary seaweeds such as agar agar, wakame, arame, nori and kombu and these can be used in soups, stews and salads, as well as recipes for Japanese cuisine. Perhaps this is one of the reasons the Japanese are so healthy?

It's good to know that cocoa powder is high in magnesium because this means that good quality chocolates are a high source of magnesium – enjoy!

Just for the fun of it, I'll close out this list of foods with 10 that contain very little or no magnesium. That's not to say they're not tasty – or that some of them are not good for you in other ways – it's just that where magnesium is concerned, their rating is very low or zero.

Honey	Radishes
Pancake syrup	Unsalted butter
Hard lollies	Italian salad dressing
Canola oil	Italian gelato, milk free
Beef broth soup	Olive oil

This list of magnesium foods on page 67-70 is far from complete. There are certainly hundreds of other foods that could have been included, many of them with significant levels of magnesium. In choosing these particular foods, I tried to offer as wide a variety as possible in the space I had available.

Just make sure that you prepare well-balanced meals, not overdoing it on any one food, and always eat in moderation.

Staying healthy means eating healthy – and eating healthy does mean getting plenty of magnesium in your diet.

On the next few pages we include some delicious and healthy recipes that contain spinach. You will remember that spinach, like all dark green leafy vegetables, is very high in magnesium.

These fabulous recipes were provided courtesy of **Audrey Tea** author of **The Sandra Cabot Recipe Collection**.

Tasty Recipes High in Magnesium

Nuts, Grains, Seeds and Greens Salad

½ cup burghal – cracked wheat

½ cup sunflower seeds

½ cup slivered almonds

1 large red or salad onion finely chopped

1 cup finely chopped spinach/silverbeet leaves

1 cup finely chopped mint

1 cup finely chopped parsley

1 cup cherry tomatoes

½ cup fresh lemon juice

½ cup cold pressed olive oil

Ground black pepper and sea salt to taste

Method

Soak burghal in 1 cup warm water for 2 hours, strain and pat dry on paper towel. Mix all ingredients together, except oil, lemon juice, salt and pepper. Lightly toss to combine, then add oil, lemon juice, salt and pepper. Cover with food wrap and refrigerate for at least 1 hour before serving to allow flavors to blend.

Quick rice side dish

2 cups cooked long grain rice (white or brown)

1 cup finely sliced celery

1 tablespoon cold pressed olive oil

2 onions, chopped

1 cup sliced mushrooms

1 teaspoon freshly chopped thyme

1½ cups shredded spinach/silverbeet

½ cup milk (dairy or unsweetened soy)

Sprinkle of chilli powder

Pepper and salt to taste

Method

Heat oil in pan and brown onions, then add celery and cook 2 – 3 mins. Add mushrooms, cook further 1 – 2 mins, add thyme and rice, mix well and keep warm. Puree the spinach and milk in a blender until smooth, add to the rice mixture, stir and heat through. Season to taste. Can be served with BBQ meats, chicken or fish.

Popeye's Spinach Soup

500 gm (16 oz) spinach or silverbeet, rinsed and trimmed

2 stems celery

2 potatoes – medium

1 tablespoon cold pressed olive oil

1 onion, chopped

4 cups dairy milk

½ cup cream

½ teaspoon ground nutmeg

Freshly ground pepper and salt to taste

Method

Peel, chop and boil potatoes until tender, drain. Cook spinach and celery in a little water until tender. Heat oil and brown onion. Blend spinach, potatoes and onion with a dash of milk and process until pureed, then add to a saucepan with all other ingredients and heat until nearly boiling. Stir often. Do not let soup bubble. Serve hot and if desired sprinkle with Parmesan cheese. Serves 4 – 6.

Not suitable to freeze.

Spinach Pie - Delicious!

3 sheets frozen short pastry

1 bunch spinach, washed and stalks removed

½ cup chopped pistachio nuts or cashews

2 tablespoons chopped raisins

3 spring onions, chopped

¼ cup grated Parmesan cheese

½ cup grated tasty cheddar cheese

4 eggs

½ cup cream

½ teaspoon allspice

Salt and ground pepper to taste

Method

Oil a 23cm (9 inch) pie dish and place 1 sheet of pastry over base; cut and join extra pieces to completely cover base. Shred and cook spinach until just tender, drain and squeeze out any extra moisture. Lightly beat eggs and retain about 2 teaspoons for brushing. Mix all ingredients together and season to taste. Pour mixture into pie dish. Lay remaining pastry over top of pie dish, joining where necessary. Pinch the edges firmly together. Pierce top of pastry in several places to allow steam to escape.

Brush with retained egg and place in a moderate oven 180°C or 356°F (or 160°C or 320°F if fan forced) and bake for about 45 mins until golden. Serve warm with salad of your choice. Serves 4 - 6.

This pie is suitable for picnic food and is also delicious cold.

Not suitable to freeze.

Spinach Slice

6 eggs, lightly beaten

½ cup milk

½ cup cream

1 red onion, finely chopped

1 teaspoon minced garlic

½ teaspoon ground nutmeg

½ teaspoon curry powder

2 tablespoons finely chopped red capsicum

1 tablespoon finely chopped parsley

¼ cup grated Parmesan cheese

½ cup grated tasty cheddar cheese

250 gm (8 oz) frozen spinach, thawed or the equivalent of fresh cooked spinach

Ground black pepper and salt to taste

Method

Whisk eggs, milk, cream and spices together. Add all other ingredients, except spinach and stir to combine. Squeeze any excess moisture from spinach and stir into mixture. Pour mixture into an oiled 23cm (9 inch) pie dish and bake in a moderate oven 180°C or 356°F (or 160°C or 320°F if fan forced) for about 30 mins or until set and lightly browned. Serve warm or cold. Cut into wedges and serve with tomato, cucumber and green leafy salad. Serves 4 -6.

Magnesium:
The Miracle Mineral

Chapter 6
Magnesium Requirements

Magnesium is extremely important for a healthy body and a healthy life – that's a fact I think we've established beyond any uncertainty or doubt. What I have not yet emphasized as strongly, however, is that magnesium is crucial during all stages of life, from infancy to old age.

In children, magnesium contributes to the proper growth of bones and teeth and is thought to help, too, with physical and mental development. Women from their teens through their late 30s or early 40s need magnesium to prevent osteoporosis later in life, while women who are pregnant at any age should take magnesium to help ensure their health and that of their babies (see **Eclampsia** in Chapter 3).

For all adults – both male and female – magnesium can help control a wide range of common ailments, from high blood pressure to high blood sugar levels (see Chapters 2-4). The result is a lower risk of many potentially deadly diseases, including heart disease and diabetes.

People past 70 tend to absorb less magnesium as it passes through their intestines, while also excreting more in their urine – so it's very important that the elderly likewise get an adequate daily dose of magnesium.

Regardless of age, your metabolic rate and your stress levels also come into play when you're determining your daily magnesium minimum, and let's not forget that men are generally going to need more magnesium than women.

Having said all of this, I guess the obvious question is now going to be, "What is the recommended daily intake of magnesium?" Based on the preceding paragraphs, the answer should probably be just as obvious, "It is going to vary."

In the opening chapters, I briefly touched on the RDA (recommended daily allowance) and RDI (recommended daily intake) of magnesium. (A reminder: RDI, which is used in Australia, is 10 percent less than the RDA used in the United States and other countries.)

Depending on your age and your sex, the current recommended RDA for magnesium is between 300 and 400 milligrams a day for adolescents and adults, less for children. It is possible, though, to be a little more specific.

What many people tend to forget when considering RDA and RDI is that these numbers are formulated to help the average healthy person achieve average magnesium levels under average circumstances. They are not designed to help you achieve optimum health, nor do they take into account the many conditions (see Chapter 1) that affect the body's ability to maintain adequate magnesium reserves or increase its need for magnesium.

Frankly, I don't believe that either the RDA or the RDI provide a sufficient amount of magnesium to meet your body's total needs – but they do give you a baseline, a starting point from which you can determine your personal magnesium requirement. You can either do this on your own – and *Magnesium: The Miracle Mineral* will certainly help in that regard – or you can seek out a nutritionist or another healthcare professional who specializes in diet, supplements and nutrition. For more information call my Health Advisory Service on +1 623 334 3232 in the USA or (02) 4655 8855 in Australia. Alternatively email ehelp@liverdoctor. com. Alternatively email ehelp@liverdoctor.com.

Either way, do keep in mind that the following magnesium guide is not gospel, just a general recommendation – and that in this particular case "mg" refers to "milligrams per day." These numbers come from a variety of sources, all of which I consider to be most reputable.

DAILY MAGNESIUM REQUIREMENTS

Age/Life Stage	Male	Female
Infants, 0-6 months	30 mg	30 mg
Infants, 7-12 months	75 mg	75 mg
Children, 1-3 years	80 mg	80 mg
Children, 4-8 years	130 mg	130 mg
Children, 9-10 years	170 mg	170 mg
Children, 11-13 years	240 mg	240 mg
Adolescents, 14-18 years	410 mg	360 mg
Adults, 19-30 years	400 mg	310 mg
Adults, 31-50 years	420 mg	320 mg
Adults, 51-70 years	420 mg	320 mg
Greater than 70 years	420 mg	320 mg
Pregnant, 18 and under	—	400 mg
Pregnant, 19-30 years	—	350 mg
Pregnant, 31 years +	—	360 mg
Breast feeding, 18 and under	—	360 mg
Breast feeding, 19-30 years	—	310 mg
Breast feeding, 31 years +	—	320 mg

Safety Issues of magnesium supplements

Any time you take a medication – prescription or over-the-counter – or even a natural supplement such as magnesium, there is going to be the possibility of an adverse reaction if you take too much, too often. Fortunately, magnesium is usually very well tolerated and the adverse effects that have been identified are related to magnesium supplements, or medications containing magnesium, and not the magnesium that occurs naturally in food.

In the average, healthy person, the most common negative effect of using excess doses of a magnesium supplement is diarrhea, with nausea and cramping being two other associated intestinal symptoms. (This is not unexpected, since one of the many therapeutic uses of magnesium is as a laxative). All of these symptoms – which typically occur with magnesium doses larger than 400 mg a day – are less likely to occur if the magnesium is taken with food and in divided doses (meaning the whole dose is not taken all at one time).

When figuring your daily magnesium dose, do keep in mind that a fairly significant number of prescription and over-the-counter medicines – some antacid and laxative products, as an example – do contain magnesium. The amount will vary although it's usually small, but you still need to factor these dosages into your magnesium calculations.

All of my research, plus my years of experience as a medical doctor, tells me that a serious overdose of magnesium is extremely rare. I myself have never seen any patients who have had significant side effects from taking a magnesium supplement. If an overdose of magnesium were to occur, as in the case of someone accidentally taking a particularly high dose of magnesium, symptoms would most likely include severe diarrhea, muscle weakness, lethargy, confusion and a slowing of breathing.

Patients with renal (kidney) failure can only take mineral supplements (including magnesium) under the supervision of their renal specialist and dietician. The risk of magnesium toxicity increases with kidney failure because the kidneys lose the ability to excrete excess magnesium from the body.

The powder form of magnesium is highly bio-available (well absorbed) and works better for those with a sensitive stomach or irritable bowel syndrome. The powder form is also quicker acting.

But again, most doctors and naturopaths will go a lifetime without ever seeing a magnesium overdose.

The one magnesium-related problem that I feel deserves special attention is the possible interaction with drugs. As an example, if you take magnesium in conjunction with some antibiotics, the magnesium may reduce the effectiveness of those antibiotics. Or, if you take magnesium and iron together at the same time, the magnesium may decrease the absorption of iron.

Drugs and Magnesium Suppliments

A partial list of the drugs, classes of drugs or supplements that may have an undesirable interaction with magnesium would include:

- Quinolones
- Antibiotics, such as the tetracycline class of antibiotics, or ciprofloxacin, nitrofurantoin, zithromax or norfloxacin antibiotics
- Lipitor – a type of statin drug used to lower cholesterol
- Certain anti-malarial drugs
- Glipizide or Glyburide
- Tagamet – anti-ulcer drug
- Calcium channel blockers – used to treat high blood pressure
- Calcium in high doses, which can fight the effect of magnesium on the muscles and arteries

Many of the possible adverse interactions from the drugs listed above would only occur if you took very high doses of magnesium. Thus the fact that you may need any of these drugs is not an absolute contraindication to taking a magnesium supplement or increasing magnesium in your diet.

For example, someone taking the drug Lipitor would have high cholesterol and/or risk factors for cardiovascular disease, so it would be a pity if they did not have the option to benefit from magnesium's life saving benefits. Just because you are taking any of the medications listed above, this does not mean that you cannot take a magnesium supplement – just check with your doctor before you start taking it.

Indeed, a significant number of patients taking statin drugs to lower cholesterol, develop problems with their muscles and ligaments, which manifests as muscle pain and weakness and increased susceptibility to tendon damage. These side effects can be permanent. To reduce the risk of side effects it is important to take supplements of magnesium and co-enzyme Q 10 whilst taking the statin drugs.

For excellent information on how to lower cholesterol levels naturally, see the book **Cholesterol – The Real Truth.**

Magnesium and Calcium

I'd like to expound just a bit on magnesium and calcium, as these two supplements need to be balanced. Not only is magnesium a key to calcium metabolism, it also protects your body from some of the undesirable effects of excess calcium, (such as muscle spasms, high blood pressure, kidney stones, poor circulation and rapid heartbeat.) As with many things in nature, balance – in this case, a balance of magnesium and calcium – is one of the hallmarks of good health.

It is best to take your magnesium supplement at a different time to any calcium supplement you may be taking.

As for the list on page 80, it is not complete. And along with mentioning these potential adverse interactions, I also need to remind you that people with kidney failure and certain types of cardiac arrythmia (such as high-grade atrio-ventricular block), should not take a magnesium supplement unless it is under a doctor's supervision.

In fact, I would recommend that anyone with a pre-existing medical problem who is considering taking magnesium in supplement form, first talk to their healthcare provider or phone my Health Advisory Service in the USA 623 334 3232 or 02 4655 8855 in Australia. Alternatively email ehelp@liverdoctor.com.

Magnesium is indeed a miracle mineral, but like many good things, the secret to enjoying the maximum benefits is judicious and regular use, not overuse. Used properly and on a regular basis, magnesium can put you on – and keep you on – the path toward a healthier and, in many cases, a longer life.

By any account, that has to qualify as a miracle.

Magnesium and athletes

The powder form of magnesium is preferred for athletes who are required to perform at top level and peak efficiency. Before the competition or match, take one flat teaspoon of an ultra potent powder form of magnesium. Some powders are available that contain magnesium mixed with taurine and selenium and sweetened with the naturally sweet herb stevia. You may need to take some extra powder several hours later, if you are competing in endurance sports.

Magnesium can certainly give you the competitive edge, as it promotes quick mental and physical energy, increases muscle strength and muscle endurance, and prevents muscle cramps.

Many elite sports people have lost a championship because they have suffered the acute onset of severe cramps during the competition - if only their coach had known about the power of magnesium to maximise performance and endurance and prevent muscle cramps.

For those folks who suffer with poor sleep and/or nocturnal cramps, it's best to take a dose of magnesium several hours before retiring to prevent these problems from occurring. You will find that you often need to increase the daily dose of magnesium in very hot weather, if you are stressed or you intend to play competitive sports.

Children and magnesium supplements

For children under the age of 9 years, it is much more preferable to use a powder form of magnesium.

Powders are available that combine magnesium with the amino acid taurine and the mineral selenium and this will help to relax the nervous system in irritable children, as well as strengthen their immune system.

The powder can be stirred into water or juice and it is easy to adjust the dose for children – for example, one can use 1/8 - 1/4 of a teaspoon of the powder daily. See the table on page 78 or call my Health Advisory Service Health Advisory Service in the USA 623 334 3232 or 02 4655 8855 in Australia. Alternatively email ehelp@liverdoctor.com. Alternatively email ehelp@liverdoctor.com.

Magnesium:
The Miracle Mineral

Chapter 7
History of Magnesium

Modern scientific studies on the relationship between magnesium and physical and mental health date back a half a century or more. And while it's true that many researchers in the mainstream medical and pharmaceutical communities have chosen to ignore the benefits of this "miracle mineral," not everyone has so easily dismissed the obvious.

As I mentioned briefly in the Introduction, magnesium is a naturally occurring element that is found in ground water and seawater, as well as in rocks and all plants and animals. It ranks fifth among the most common minerals in the earth's crust and, according to at least one report, has been used for its therapeutic benefits – including the use of magnesium salts in spas – for 2,000 years or longer.

Most written history of magnesium dates to 18th century England, when a farmer (his name is lost in the pages of history) in the community of Epsom tried to give his cows water from a well, only to have them turn up their noses and refuse to drink it. This led to the farmer's discovery that the water had a somewhat bitter taste. The fact that the farmer and his family then chose to use the water themselves leads me to suppose that they were less particular than their cows.

At any rate, the farmer eventually discovered that his well water seemed to heal rashes and small cuts. As word of this natural remedy spread, the farmer began to receive widespread recognition for his discovery – which became known as "Epsom salt." In this homeopathic, pre-antibiotic era, anything with healing properties was eagerly welcomed, so the farmer's fame is certainly understandable. Scientists would later discover that the key ingredient in Epsom salt was magnesium sulphate.

If we fast-forward 50 years or so, to 1808, we have Sir Humphrey Davy isolating the magnesium element in Epsom salt and concocting a mixture of magnesia. According to most published reports, Davy initially planned to name the newly isolated element "magnium," but for a reason I've not been able to determine, he instead used "magnesium." This is said to come from the Greek word "Magnesia," which was a city and a district of Thessaly where magnesium was apparently recorded as a component of soapstone.

In the two centuries since Davy helped open the doors to the beneficial world of magnesium and laid the groundwork for future research, much has been learned about this wonderful mineral. Foremost is the importance of magnesium to a healthy mind and body and the many mental and physical problems that may occur when a deficiency is present.

Research has also revealed that the best way to get the magnesium our bodies need is by following a healthy diet. For instance, eating a daily variety of whole grains, legumes and vegetables – particularly dark-green, leafy vegetables – is a good way to both ensure that you are getting your recommended daily allowance of magnesium and to help your body make up any small, pre-existing diet-related deficiency.

Some people receive additional magnesium in their medications. Some antacids contain magnesium, as do some laxatives and anticonvulsant and anti-inflammatory drugs, as well as other types of over-the-counter and prescription drugs. But within the context of preventing or reversing a magnesium deficiency, these sources are generally insignificant.

The reason a proper diet that includes a lot of magnesium-laden foods is so important is that if you allow your magnesium levels to drop too low, then simply "increasing dietary intake of magnesium may not be enough to restore ... magnesium levels to normal." This is according to the National Institutes of Health (NIH), a branch of the United States government. When diet alone is not sufficient to boost your magnesium levels into the normal range, a magnesium supplement is required.

Fortunately, there are quite a few supplements available on today's market, in pharmacies and in health food stores.

Unfortunately, not all magnesium supplements are created equal – see page 88.

– see page 88.

Magnesium Deficiency or Depletion?

There are essentially two different routes by which you can end up magnesium deficient.

1. Magnesium Deficiency

"Magnesium deficiency" is actually defined as a disorder that corresponds to an insufficient intake of magnesium.

By "insufficient intake," I mean that you are eating too many unhealthy foods (such as processed and refined sugary foods, and/or refined white flour and foods that are high in processed hydrogenated fat) that not only don't contain much, if any, magnesium, but can also deplete your body's existing supply. And you are not eating enough of the healthy foods that do provide magnesium.

2. Magnesium Depletion

There is a second and **more serious condition** known as "magnesium depletion," which is caused by poor absorption or loss of magnesium. This is a disorder that, in general, is caused by a malfunction of the control mechanisms that regulate your body's magnesium levels. In other words, your body is prevented from using the magnesium that you ingest in food.

Dietary magnesium is absorbed from the small intestines and then transported in the blood to the cells and tissues where it is needed. Causes of magnesium depletion range from stomach and intestinal disorders such as Crohn's disease, celiac disease, intestinal surgery and vomiting and diarrhea. Healthy, normal kidneys are able to reduce the excretion of magnesium in people with low magnesium levels in their blood; however, if kidney disease is present this may be impaired.

Excess loss of magnesium in the urine can occur with poorly controlled diabetes and alcohol abuse. Some medications increase the loss of magnesium in the urine. The most dangerous medications to cause this problem are strong diuretic drugs and drugs which block the production of hydrochloric acid in the stomach. If magnesium levels become very low, dangerous cardiac arrythmias may occur.

Magnesium depletion is a serious problem that demands professional treatment. In some cases, high magnesium doses must be given intravenously to help you reach an optimum level.

If you suspect that magnesium depletion may be the cause of your health problems, then I would definitely recommend that you put yourself under the care of a medical professional and do not attempt to treat yourself without help.

The purpose of **Magnesium: The Miracle Mineral** is not to replace proper and adequate medical care for people suffering with magnesium depletion or malabsorption. Rather, my goal in writing this book is to spread the word as far and as wide as possible about the many different health benefits of magnesium, while helping people who have a diet-related deficiency make sure they are getting an adequate daily dosage of this very important – indeed, life enhancing and potentially life saving – mineral.

Having said this, I'll now return to using "magnesium deficiency" as the catch-all phrase to describe the common condition in which you have a less than desirable daily intake of magnesium, that results in abnormally low levels of total body magnesium.

As a reminder, the current RDA (recommended daily allowance) is between 300 and 400 milligrams (mg) a day, depending on your age and your sex. Some doctors and nutritionists chart the RDA as high as 450 mg a day, and the difference is slight enough, and the mineral important enough, that I wouldn't argue with that figure. In Australia, the RDI (recommended daily intake) is the standard, though you'll recall that the RDI is 10 percent less than the RDA used in the United States and other countries.

It's a fact that individuals do vary widely in their magnesium needs, and some researchers in the field have found that women, on average, need less magnesium than men.

If you feel healthy most of the time, regularly eat many of the foods that I list in Chapter 5, have none of the conditions listed in Chapter 1 that can lead to a magnesium deficiency, and likewise have none of the deficiency symptoms from Chapter 1, then congratulations! You may be one of the relatively few people who are maintaining a healthy level of magnesium.

Magnesium Supplements

Most people, however, truly don't get an adequate amount of magnesium on a daily basis. "Well, I come close," you might say, "so I'm not too concerned." You should be concerned, though. When it comes to meeting your body's magnesium requirements, "close" is never going to be good enough.

Consider this: If your body requires 400 mg of magnesium a day, but you're only getting an average of 390 mg, then you're coming up short by 10 mg a day. That 10 mg seems almost insignificant, so if you were aware of these numbers you'd probably be inclined to say, "No big deal ... 10 milligrams, that's only 2.5 percent of my daily requirement."

But it is a big deal, because there's the big picture to consider.

You'd be right in thinking that a one-time magnesium shortage of 10 mg is nothing to worry about. But in a week's time you would be coming up short by 70 mg, and over a year's time you're looking at a shortage of more than 3,600 mg. That equals a nine-day supply based on a 400mg daily requirement.

You have to look at the cumulative effect when considering magnesium loss – and I can assure you that for most people, their daily negative loss is much greater than 10 mg. That's why supplements do have an important role in establishing our magnesium balance.

Eating a healthy diet is important for many reasons other than magnesium intake. We all know that. But if you feel that for whatever reason your dietary intake of magnesium is insufficient, a magnesium supplement may be the key to improving your well being.

For most of us, these supplements will be taken in oral form, which, as I've mentioned, are readily available from a variety of sources. In talking to some of my patients, though, I've found that it's not uncommon to be undecided on the best type of supplement to take – and this even applies to people who have educated themselves on magnesium supplementation. Part of the problem is the many different formulations in which magnesium is used.

As an example, the types of magnesium supplements available are:

Magnesium oxide, magnesium carbonate, magnesium hydroxide, magnesium phosphate, magnesium amino acid chelate, magnesium glycinate, magnesium citrate, magnesium lactate, magnesium chloride, magnesium sulphate, magnesium aspartate, magnesium orotate, magnesium ascorbate and magnesium gluconate.

Among the things you also need to consider when choosing a supplement are:

- Magnesium content (amount of the pure mineral magnesium) – this is also known as the elemental magnesium content in a supplement

- Bioavailability (the ability of the magnesium to be absorbed into the blood stream and inside the cells)

Oral supplements combine magnesium with other substances, such as salt, and the **actual amount of magnesium** does vary greatly from supplement to supplement. To demonstrate, see the list below

Magnesium oxide	60 percent magnesium
Magnesium carbonate	45 percent magnesium
Magnesium hydroxide	42 percent magnesium
Magnesium phosphate	21 percent magnesium
Magnesium amino acid chelate	20 percent magnesium
Magnesium glycinate	18 percent magnesium
Magnesium citrate	16 percent magnesium
Magnesium lactate	12 percent magnesium
Magnesium chloride	12 percent magnesium
Magnesium sulphate	10 percent magnesium
Magnesium aspartate	6.7 percent magnesium
Magnesium orotate	6.5 percent magnesium
Magnesium ascorbate	6.0 percent magnesium

The percentage of pure (or elemental) magnesium contained in a supplement is relevant because, as a rule, magnesium supplements are poorly absorbed – which is what bioavailability is all about. The NIH defines bioavailability as *"the amount of magnesium in food, medications and supplements that is absorbed by the intestines and ultimately available for biological activity in your cells and tissues."*

To further confuse the issue, a study cited by the NIH found that just because a given supplement has a high elemental magnesium content, this doesn't automatically mean that taking it will result in your body absorbing more magnesium.

The study compared four forms of magnesium preparations, with the results showing lower bioavailability of magnesium oxide – which has a magnesium content of 60 percent – and higher bioavailability of magnesium chloride and magnesium lactate – each with only a 12 percent magnesium content.

I have found that the better absorbed forms of magnesium are – magnesium phosphate, magnesium aspartate, magnesium orotate, magnesium glycinate and magnesium amino acid chelate. In particular, the orotate form of magnesium is better at transporting the magnesium ion inside the cells where it is needed. The amino acid chelate form and the aspartate form are highly bioavailable.

It is worth mentioning here too, that if magnesium is being used to combat panic attacks, palpitations, epilepsy or severe muscle spasms, it is possible to get a better effect in reducing these problems by taking a powder form of magnesium that also contains the amino acid taurine. Taurine, like magnesium, stabilizes the electrical potential across cell membranes, which augments the preventative effect of magnesium in these conditions.

In my opinion, it is generally best to take a complete form of magnesium that combines several different types of magnesium all in one tablet or all in one powder.

Magnesium Complete tablets contain 5 different types of magnesium all in one tablet. Each tablet contains magnesium orotate, magnesium citrate, magnesium chelate, magnesium aspartate and magnesium phosphate. See www.liverdoctor. com or phone 623 334 3232 in the USA or 02 4655 8855 in Australia and speak to one of our naturopaths.

Both the powder and the tablet forms are effective in increasing body magnesium levels but the powder is faster absorbed and thus is quicker acting.

There are so many choices

In spite of all these differences, some self-proclaimed experts in the field will tell you that it doesn't matter significantly which form of magnesium you use, or whether you take your daily supplement all at once or at several different times during the day. Personally, I don't agree with either of these opinions.

There is a difference between supplements!

Magnesium oxide, for instance, is commonly available and cheap, but can be difficult to digest and absorb. In my experience magnesium oxide more commonly causes digestive upsets probably because it is poorly absorbed.

Trying to increase your magnesium intake with a multivitamin-mineral tablet only will not be enough. It is essential to take a magnesium supplement that is dedicated to providing you with a good dose of magnesium in a well absorbed form.

In particular, it is not as effective to take a supplement that combines magnesium with calcium, because these two minerals exert opposite effects on the blood vessels. Calcium causes the blood vessels to constrict and that is why "calcium blocker drugs" are used to treat high blood pressure. Magnesium causes the blood vessels to relax and dilate, which is opposite to the effect of calcium. Thus, if you take high doses of calcium and magnesium at the same time, they will fight each other.

Furthermore, magnesium can reduce the undesirable build up of excess calcium in the arteries, urinary tract and soft tissues; this is another reason that it is not desirable to take a magnesium supplement that contains calcium.

How to take magnesium

Regardless of the supplement you choose, I'd suggest taking it in several smaller doses throughout the day, or at least twice daily, as opposed to one large dose. For instance, if you want to supplement your diet with an additional 400 mg of magnesium a day, try two doses of 200 mg each, instead of taking the entire 400 mg all at once.

For most people however, there is no problem taking the whole dose at once and it's better than forgetting to take it. Some find that the magnesium works better in divided doses. Still others find that if the whole dose is taken all at once an unwanted laxative effect may occur.

You can always start off with a single dose of approximately 100 mg to 200 mg, see how your stomach reacts and then adjust your dosage if necessary. I also suggest taking any magnesium supplement with food, although if you forget, it's fine to take it with a glass of water only.

If you find that magnesium tablets upset your digestive system, I recommend that you try a powder form – start with only ¼ of a flat teaspoon daily in water or juice, then gradually build up the dose so that you can take ½ teaspoon once or twice daily.

References

Seelig, Mildred S., M.D., MPH, Rosanoff, Andrea, Ph.D., The Magnesium Factor. New York: Avery, a member of Penguin Group (USA) Inc., 2003.

Murray, Michael, N.D., Pizzorno, Joseph, N.D., Encyclopedia of Natural Medicine. Revised 2nd Edition. New York: Three Rivers Press, 1998.

Thomas, Clayton L., M.D., Editor. Taber's Cyclopedic Medical Dictionary. Edition 18. Philadelphia: F.A. Davis Company, 1997.

U.S. Department of Agriculture, Agricultural Research Service, 2001. USDA Nutrient Database for Standard Reference, Release 14.

Kozielec, T., Starobrat-Hermelin, B. Assessment of magnesium levels in children with attention deficit hyperactivity disorder (ADHD). Magnes Res. 1997 June; 10(2): 143-8

Maier, J.A. Low magnesium and atherosclerosis: an evidence-based link. Mol Aspects Med. 2003 Feb-Jun; 24(1-3): 137-46.

Cheung, Anthony C.S., Goyal, Naresh, Magnesium. Journal of the Hong Kong Medical Association, Vol. 37, No. 4, 1985.

Skotnicki, A.B., Jablonski, M.J., Musial, J., Swadzba, J. The role of magnesium in the pathogenesis and therapy of bronchial asthma. Przegl Lek. 1997; 54(9): 630-3.

Goggs, R., Vaughan-Thomas, A., et al. Nutraceutical therapies for degenerative joint diseases: a critical review. Crit Rev Food Sci Nutr. 2005: 45(3): 145-64

Lietzmann, C. Vegetarian diets: what are the advantages? Forum Nutr. 2005; (57): 147-56

Eby, G.A., Eby, K.L. Rapid recovery from major depression using magnesium treatment. Medical Hypothesis. 2006 March 14.

Kinnunen, O., Salokannel, J. Constipation is elderly long-stay patients: its treatment by magnesium hydroxide and bulk-laxative. Ann Clin Res. 1987; 19(5): 321-3.

Seelig, M.S., M.D. Inter-relationship of magnesium and congestive heart failure. Wien Med Wochenschr. 2000; 150(15-16): 335-41.

Werbach, Melvyn, M.D. Treating chronic fatigue syndrome by repleting mineral deficiencies. Journal of the Australasian College of Nutritional and Environmental Medicine. December 2004, page 15.

Holdcraft, L.C., Assefi, N., Buchwald, D. Complementary and alternative medicine in fibromyalgia and related syndromes. Best Pract Res Clin Rheumatol. 2003 Aug; 17(4): 667-83.

Sarac, A.J., Gur, A. Complementary and alternative medical therapies in fibromyalgia. Curr Pharm Des. 2006; 12(1): 47-57.

Head, K.A. Natural therapies for ocular disorders, part two: cataracts and glaucoma. Altern Med Rev. 2001 Apr; 6(2): 141-66.

Gazpar, A.Z., Gasser, P., Flammer, J. The influence of magnesium on visual field and peripheral vasospasm in glaucoma. Ophthalmologica. 1995; 209(1): 11-3.

Hornyak, M., et al. Magnesium therapy for periodic leg movements-related insomnia and restless legs syndrome: an open pilot study. Sleep. 1998 Aug 1; 21(5): 501-5.

Yasui, M., Ota, K. Experimental and clinical studies on dysregulation of magnesium metabolism in the aetiopathogenesis of multiple sclerosis. Magnes. Res. 1992 Dec; 5(4): 295-302.

Rossier, P., van Erven, S., Wade, D.T. The effects of magnesium oral therapy on spasticity in a patient with multiple sclerosis. Eur J Neruol. 2000 Nov; 7(6): 741-4.

Mauskop, A., Altura, B.M. Role of magnesium in the pathogenesis and treatment of migraines. Clin Neurosci. 1998; 5(1): 24-7.

Teo, K.K., Yusuf, S. Role of magnesium in reducing mortality in acute myocardial infarction, A review of the evidence. Drugs. 1993; 46: 347-59.

Turlapaty, P.D.M.V., Altura, B.M. Magnesium deficiency produces spasms of coronary arteries: Relationship to etiology of sudden death ischemic heart disease. Sci. 1980; 208: 199-200.

Witteman, J.C.M., et al. Reduction of blood pressure with oral magnesium supplementation in women with mild to moderate hypertension. Am Jour Clin Nutr. 1994; 60: 129-35.

Altura, B.M., Altura, B.T. Tension headaches and muscle tension: Is there a role for magnesium? Med Hypotheses. 2001 Dec; 57(6): 705-13.

Roffe, C., Sills, S., Crome, P., Jones, P. Randomized, cross-over controlled trial of magnesium citrate in the treatment of chronic persistent leg cramps. Med Sci Monit. 2002 May; 8(5): CR326-30.

Johnson, S. The multifaceted and widespread pathology of magnesium deficiency. Med Hypotheses. 2001 Feb; 56(2): 163-70.

Takahashi, H., et al. A case of chronic fatigue syndrome who showed a beneficial effect by intravenous administration of magnesium sulphate. Arerugi. 1992 Nov; 41(11): 1605-10.

Yu-Yahiro, J.A. Electrolytes and their relationship to normal and abnormal muscle function. Orthop Nurs. 1194 Sep-Oct; 13(5): 38-40.

Olerich, M.A., Rude, R.K. Should we supplement magnesium in critically ill patients? New Horiz. 1994 May; 2(2): 186-92.

Kiss, S.A., Dombovari, J., Oncsik, M. Magnesium inhibits the harmful effects on plants of some toxic elements. Magnes Res. 1991 Mar: 4(1): 3-7.

Yasui, M., Kihira, T. Ota, K. Calcium, magnesium and aluminum concentrations in Parkinson's disease. Neurotoxicology. 1992 Fall; 13(3): 593-600.

Golts, N., et al. Magnesium inhibits spontaneous and iron-induced aggregation of alpha-synuclein. J Biol Chem. 2002 May; 277(18): 16116-23.

Schecter, M., et al. Effects of oral magnesium therapy on exercise tolerance, exercise-induced chest pain and quality of life in patients with coronary artery disease. American Journal of Cardiology. 2003; 91: 517-21.

Hall, A. Magnesium and cardiovascular disease. Bioceuticals. 2000; Vol 17.

Magnesium: widespread benefits. Albion Research Notes. 1992 Sept: Vol. 2, No. 2.

Magnesium: clinical and health benefits still without limits. Albion Research Notes. 2003 Oct. Vol. 12, No. 3.

Caddell, J.L. Magnesium deficiency promotes muscle weakness, contributing to the risk of sudden infant death (SIDS) in infants sleeping prone. Magnes Res. 2001 Mar; 14 (1-2): 39-50.

Online References

Asthma and magnesium deficiency. www.mgwater.com/asthma.shtml

Magnesium. www.krispin.com/magnes.html

Highest magnesium foods. http://wij.fre.fr/magnes.txt

Magnesium products. www.allergyresearchgroup.com

ADD and ADHD. www.swiftweb.com/ha/book2.html

What is magnesium and what does it do? www.nysopep.org/page.cfm/67

Magnesium metabolism. www.merck.com

Present and future of magnesium research. www.mgwater.com/dur05.shtml

The history of magnesium. www.academic.greensboroday.org

Magnesium. www.dietary-supplements.info.nih.gov

Magnesium. www.pdrhealth.com

Chronic fatigue. www.mgwater.com/chroniclz.shtml

Magnesium deficiency and ADD. www.vpr.com/art/1634.asp

Naturopathic perspectives. Approaches to anxiety. www.townsendletter.com

The importance of magnesium. www.eidon.com/magnesium_article.htm

Using calcium and magnesium for constipation. www.alumbo.com

Oral magnesium for cardiac arrhythmias. www.mgwater.com/arr.shtml

Rapid recovery from major depression using magnesium treatment.
www.intl.elsevierhealth.com

The miracle of magnesium.
www.mercola.com/2004/aug/7/miracle_magnesium.htm

Magnesium and magnesium deficiency. www.audiblox2000.com

BBD supplements explained (multiple sclerosis). www.msrc.co.uk

Mitral valve prolapse: The links to magnesium deficiency. www.ctds.info

Easing symptoms of a troubled heart. www.mgwater.com/prev1808.shtml

Intercellular magnesium and Parkinson's disease. www.biosciences.utoledo.edu

Stopping the squeeze (leg cramps). www.mothernature.com

IV magnesium and stroke case study #1. www.pannaturopathic.com

Magnesium and stroke recovery. www.allbusiness.com

Mutual aggravation of magnesium and stress. www.findarticles.com

Magnesium. www.whofoods.com

Magnesium facts. www.beta-glucan-info.com

Magnesium. www.lpi.oregonstate.edu/infocenter/minerals/magnesium/index.html

Magnesium. www.preventivehealthtoday.com

Magnesium: The forgotten mineral. www.mineralresourcesint.com

Magnesium – a forgotten mineral. www.vitamintrader.com

Magnesium: The stress reliever. www.healthy.net

Health benefits of magnesium. www.wholehealthmd.com

Magnesium content of foods - U.S. Department of Agriculture's Nutrient Database
Web site: http://www.nal.usda.gov/fnic/cgi-bin/nut_search.pl.

This is what you will find at:

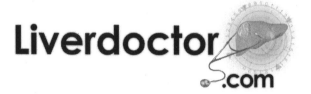

Holistic medical information

Well researched and up-to-date information to help you in your daily life
Informative on-line information to assist you look after your health and weight

Free liver check up test

Take this liver check up and receive private & confidential feedback on
the state of your liver and general health - www.liverdoctor.com/liver-check

Health supplements

Including Doctor Cabot's Livatone Plus capsules to support optimal liver function

On-line shopping

Sandra Cabot MD has a excellent range of health products and publications

On-line help from Dr Cabot's Team

Confidential and expert help from Dr Cabot's highly trained nutritionists and
naturopaths. Simply email us at ehelp@liverdoctor.com

Free LIVERISH newsletter

Register on-line for the free LIVERISH nesletter at www.liverdoctor.com/newsletter

Love you liver and live longer

www.liverdoctor.com